The OMEGA-3 Miracle

The Icelandic Longevity Secret that Offers
Super Protection Against Heart Disease, Cancer, Diabetes,
Arthritis, Premature Aging, and Deadly Inflammation

by Garry Gordon, M.D., D.O., M.D.(H.)

and

Herb Joiner-Bey, N.D.

Disclaimer: This information is presented by independent
medical experts whose sources of information include studies from the world's medical and scientific literature, patient
records, and other clinical and anecdotal reports. The
material in this book is for informational purposes only
and is not intended for the diagnosis or treatment of
disease. Please visit a medical health professional for
specific diagnosis of any ailments mentioned or discussed
in this material.

Book design by Bonnie Lambert

ISBN 1-893910-34-2
Seventeenth printing
Published by Freedom Press
1801 Chart Trail
Topanga, CA 90290
Bulk Orders Available: (800) 959-9797
E-mail: info@freedompressonline.com

PRINTED IN THE USA

Contents

Introduction: The Icelandic Longevity Secret   5

Part I—The Healing Power of OMEGA-3s
Chapter 1: Omega-3s: The Most Vital Nutrient Missing from Your Diet   *11*
Chapter 2: Overfed and Undernourished—Omega-3 Fatty Acid Deficiency—
    A Major Cause of Disease   *25*

Part II—OMEGA-3s and Your Health
Chapter 1: Omega-3s for a Healthy Heart   *37*
Chapter 2: Reduce Cancer Risk with Omega-3 Fatty Acids   *48*
Chapter 3: Omega-3s for Mental Health   *62*
Chapter 4: Omega-3s—Rescuing ADHD Children & Adults   *71*
Chapter 5: Omega-3s & Pregnancy Outcome   *87*
Chapter 6: Omega-3s—Diabetes & Omega-3s   *94*
Chapter 7: Female Health: Omega-3s to the Rescue   *101*
Chapter 8: Arthritis—A Remedy with Omega-3 Oils   *108*
Chapter 9: Omega-3s & Asthma   *114*
Chaper 10: Oil Gets In Your Eyes   *120*
Chapter 11: Weight Loss with Omega-3 Oils   *122*
Chapter 12: Flaxseed Oil—The Vegetarian Omega-3 Choice   *124*
Chapter 13: Caveat Emptor: Savvy Shopping Tips for Omega-3 Oils   *128*
Chapter 14: Putting It All Together   *133*

Appendixes:
Appendix A: Letter from Executive Office of the President of
    the United States on Omega-3s   *138*
Appendix B: Resources   *142*
Appendix C: Prescription Pain Relievers vs. Fish Oils for Osteoarthritis   *146*
Appendix D: The Beauty of Omega-3   *156*

References   *165*
Index   *173*
About the Authors   *176*

Introduction

ICELANDIC FISH OILS

In the icy North Atlantic waters lives an island nation of people who have endured the challenges of harsh weather, rugged terrain and long seasons of darkness for over one thousand years. These are the people of Iceland.

Today, Icelanders are a medical marvel. They have less heart disease, high blood pressure and stroke than any other nationality in the world. In fact, they are 20 times more likely to live longer than Americans. Studies show they live these extra years in fine

Country	Life Expectancy at Birth (years, 1990-99) Female/Male	Life Expectancy at Birth (years, 1990-99) Combined	Infant Mortality Rate (per 1,000 births, 1990-99)
Iceland	81/77	79.0	5
Italy	81/75	78.0	7
Israel	80/76	78.0	8
France	82/74	78.0	6
United Kingdom	80/75	77.5	7
Germany	80/74	77.0	5
U.S.A.	80/73	76.5	7

Source: Statistics and indicators are provided by the United Nations Statistics Division from the World Statistics Pocketbook and Statistical Yearbook, except capital cities and languages.

health, experiencing the greatest measures of happiness and contentment.

Furthermore, Iceland has the lowest rate of infant mortality. Icelandic women give birth to the healthiest infants having possibly the most advanced immune and nervous systems, with optimum brain and eye development.

What is it about the remarkable longevity of Icelanders that the rest of the world can learn from? What is their secret to living longer, healthier lives than anyone else?

Major scientific research conducted in the 1970s first identified certain fatty acids in fish found near Iceland that had remarkable healthful benefits. In 1982, a landmark study, conducted by a team of Scandinavian scientists, earned them the Nobel Prize for their discoveries of the workings of these substances.

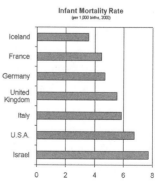

Infant Mortality Rate
(per 1,000 births, 2000)

The essence of what they discovered is something that you and all of your loved ones can take advantage of every day to live longer and healthier lives.

According to the Icelandic Longevity Institute, the daily intake of fish oils—unusually rich in essential fatty acids EPA (eicosapentaenoic acid) and DHA (docosahexaenoic acid)—is unique to Icelanders. It starts with small children and continues with even the oldest adults. The Icelandic Longevity Institute has scientific studies from around the world that show how EPA and DHA have a profound impact on maintaining good health and helping to prevent and control serious health disorders, including heart disease, cardiovascular disease, cancerous tumors, and numerous autoimmune and inflammatory diseases. Key findings include:

- EPA & DHA—Essential for good health. EPA is necessary to create prostaglandins to promote superior cardiovascular health and optimal cell membrane formation. DHA is vital for proper development and functioning of the brain, eyes, and autoimmune system.
- Promotes arterial flexibility—Omega-3 fatty acids promote the flexibility and elasticity of coronary arteries. Without omega-3, artery walls can become hard, with microscopic cracks and pockets that can become receptacles for life-threatening cholesterol.
- Fights joint disease—Omega-3 fatty acids maintain cell and joint suppleness, even decreasing pain and tenderness and the need for anti-inflammatory drugs.
- Increases brain function—Omega-3s promote neurotransmission in the brain and increase intellectual capacity.
- Positive effect on cholesterol—Omega-3s help increase high-density lipoproteins (HDLs, the "good" cholesterol), and decrease low-density lipoproteins (LDLs, the "bad" cholesterol).
- Lowered triglycerides—No other natural compound to date seems to be more effective than omega-3 to lower triglycerides, a major risk factor for heart disease.
- Reduced risk of blood clots—Omega-3s lower fibrinogen, which converts to fibrin, the main component of blood clots and thrombi, which can cause heart disease.
- Lowered chance of heart attack—Lipoprotein(a) which contributes to myocardial infarction is markedly reduced by intake of omega-3s.
- Recommended for diabetics—Omega-3 fish oils provide all these positive benefits without risk of increasing blood sugar.
- Fights signs of aging—Skin is one of the fastest reproducing cell networks in the body and needs omega-3 fatty acids to replenish and maintain the optimum cellular moisture balance. Without these essential fatty acids, skin cells age prematurely.

The healthful benefits of omega-3, also known as polyunsaturated fatty acids (PUFA), have been shown to increase the longer you take it. The recommended intake is approximately 1,000 mg daily, but higher doses can be taken for the treatment of specific disease problems upon the direction of your health advisor.

Icelanders are living proof of the importance of omega-3 fatty acids. According to an article by Richard C. Morais, entitled "Who are the happiest people?" (*Forbes*; Oct 23rd 1995), Icelanders "have the world's lowest infant mortality rate, and are fantastically long-lived."

Even more, it's been found that Icelanders are remarkably free of depression, unlike many other northern nations. According to an article by Ruut Veenhoven, entitled "Happy life expectancy—A comprehensive measure of quality of life in nations" (*Social Indicators Research*; Number 39, 1996), "The top three happiest nations [are] Sweden, the Netherlands, and at the top of the league, Iceland." Omega-3s have been clinically proven to prevent the onset of depression.

Over the last century, Icelanders started commercially producing the essential fatty acids that have been in their diet for hundreds of years. They depend on this locally processed fish oil to maintain their historical nutritional needs now that fish is too expensive for them to eat on a daily basis. You'll find their fish oil products in every cupboard in Iceland. Whereas American and European diets lack the essential fatty acids found in oily, fatty fish—in fact, they consume omega-6 fats, which are found in most cooking oils and meats and linked to heart disease and other chronic ailments, far out of proportion to omega-3s—Icelanders have maintained their historically correct omega-3 intake (close to 3 to 1, omega-6s to omega-3s) and, hence, their good health.

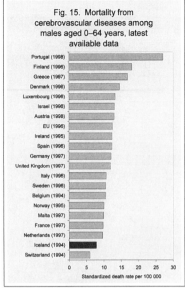

Fig. 15. Mortality from cerebrovascular diseases among males aged 0–64 years, latest available data

Data for Iceland are 3-year moving averages
Source: *Highlights on Health in Iceland*, WHO Regional Office for Europe, 2000

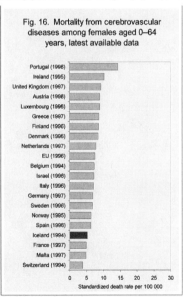

Fig. 16. Mortality from cerebrovascular diseases among females aged 0–64 years, latest available data

Data for Iceland are 3-year moving averages
Source: *Highlights on Health in Iceland*, WHO Regional Office for Europe, 2000

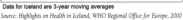

We hope you will enjoy learning about this Icelandic longevity secret.

Sincerely,

—*Garry Gordon, M.D., D.O., M.D.(H.),*
Herb Joiner-Bey, N.D.

Part I–
The Healing Power
of Omega-3s

Omega-3s: The Most Vital Nutrient Missing from Your Diet

There's a lot of good news these days about omega-3 fatty acids. In fact, the news is so good that, as physicians, we think everyone ought to be taking advantage of the omega-3s, incorporating much more of these good fats into their diets.

Even many of our colleagues—very mainstream doctors at major hospitals and university medical schools—are expounding the virtues of omega-3 fatty acids to their patients, family, friends, and the news media. Most recently, the American Heart Association altered its healthy heart dietary guidelines to recommend that foods rich in omega-3 fatty acids be consumed at least twice a week. According to the World Health Organization, omega-3 fatty acids are essential to optimal health and life. Unfortunately, almost all of our patients are sadly lacking in these essential nutrients when they visit our offices.

Omega-3 fatty acids have been traditionally supplied in the diet by wild cold-water ocean fish (herring, cod liver, salmon, mackerel, sardines, anchovies, black cod, albacore tuna) whose original food source is at the bottom of the food chain in the form of phytoplankton. "If the tissues of ocean deep water fish did not contain such a large amount of omega-3 fatty acids, they would become stiff and would not survive in the very cold water," says Dr. Tom Saldeen, professor and chairman at the Department of Forensic Medicine at the medical facility of Uppsala, Sweden and one of the world's leading experts on the health benefits of fish oils.

Omega-3 fatty acids also keep cells supple and flexible in Man, helping to maintain joint suppleness and skin and blood vessel elasticity. Such supple, flexible cells are said to be signs of youth. Omega-3 fatty acids are important constituents of the cell walls, and determine physiological properties of cell walls such as fluidity (plasticity). This depends primarily on the structure of the fatty acids. Saturated fatty acids have a straight structure, whereas omega-3 fatty acids such as (EPA) eicosapentaenoic acid and (DHA) docosahexaenoic acid are markedly curved. Saturated, straight fatty acids are packed closely together in the cell wall, which becomes stiff. Curved fatty acids such as EPA and DHA cannot be packed so closely they take up more space and therefore make the cell walls more elastic and less stiff.

Other good omega-3 sources include flaxseed, nuts and various seeds, green leafy vegetables, sea vegetables, wild game, and free-range livestock animals grazing on green vegetation (rather than being fed corn).

MOST OF US SUFFER FROM A DEFICIENCY OF FISH FATTY ACIDS (OMEGA-3 FATTY ACIDS)

Unfortunately, ocean pollution, diminishing populations of cold-water fish rich in omega-3s, and the advent of industrialized mass food production and refining of supermarket food has affected the delicate polyunsaturated omega-3 fatty acids, such that they are either destroyed, transformed to potentially toxic compounds, or deliberately removed to avoid spoilage and shelf-life.

"Our intake of different fats has changed markedly during the last century," says Dr. Saldeen. "We eat much more saturated fats and vegetable oils containing omega-6 fatty acids today, whereas our intake of fish fatty acids (omega-3) has decreased by 80 percent during the last 80 years. In the old days, it was not uncommon for fish to be eaten seven days a week. Some people working on Swedish farms tire of it, asking for a note in their employment contracts stating that salmon would not be served more than five days a week. We eat much less fish today, so most of us now suffer from a deficiency of omega-3 fatty acids. This may be of great physiological importance, especially in relation to an increased incidence of cardiovascular disease and other disease states. To keep up with the needs for fish fatty acids, we should eat 100 grams daily of fatty fish such as mackerel, herring or salmon."

As essential nutrients, omega-3 fatty acids cannot be manufactured within our bodies from other kinds of fatty acids. They must be obtained from the foods we eat. The problem is that we simply do not get enough omega-3s in our standard American diet. According to Dr. Artemis Simopoulos, M.D., author of *The Omega Diet* (HarperCollins, 1999), omega-3 fatty acids are undetectable in blood samples of 20 percent of Americans. As for the rest of us, we are critically deficient in this vital nutrient. Since the body cannot make its own omega-3 fatty acids, the need to include more omega-3 sources in our diet and to supplement our diet with rich sources of omega-3 fatty acids is great. In fact, Donald Rudin, M.D., in his book *Omega-3 Oils* (Avery, 1996) likens today's rampant omega-3 fatty acid deficiency to the classic B-vitamin deficiency diseases pellagra and beriberi of the early 1900s.

Thus, better dietary choices as well as nutritional supplementation of these vital nutrients is often imperative. Fortunately, natural fish oil is by far one of the best-documented natural pharmaceutical and food supplements available today. Says Dr. Saldeen, "During a recent ten-month period, 293 articles about fish oil were published in well-known medical journals, compared with six articles concerning *Ginkgo biloba* and 16 about ginseng. The effect of natural stable fish oil has been proven in many different scientific studies [see our references]. In these studies, the stable fish oil was given to patients for up to eight years without any adverse effects or loss of beneficial effects. Most studies were randomized, with a double-blind crossover design, meaning that the participants were assigned to different groups by lot; the same person was given active oil and placebo oil during different periods, and neither the participants nor the researchers knew the identity of the oil."

So, with both omega-3 fatty acids, we're talking about major league research, which should be reassuring to even the most skeptical readers.

DIFFERENT KINDS OF OMEGA-3 FATTY ACIDS

The two most common sources of omega-3s are cold-water fish and flaxseed (*Linium usitatissimum*). Each provides different types of omega-3 fatty acids. Flaxseed provides the omega-3 fatty acid alpha-linolenic acid (ALA), which is thought to be the parent compound of all omega-3s. Some types of cold-water fish provide two other kinds, eicosapentaenoic acid (EPA) and docosahexaenoic acid (DHA).

As we mentioned, the ALA in flaxseed is considered to be the parent compound of all omega-3 fatty acids, since it can be converted to eicosapentaneoic and docosahexaenoic acids, which help maintain healthy joints, heart functions and healthy circulation. However, sometimes this conversion in the human body is hampered by dietary practices, environmental influences, and even genetics. Both kinds of omega-3 fatty acids are important to human health. One is not superior to the other. They are simply different, and you will want both oceanic and terrestrial sources of omega-3 fatty acids in your daily fare.

Critically important, however, is the role that preformed DHA and EPA, found in some types of seafood, play in brain development. Studies on rats and rhesus monkeys reveal that dietary restriction of these omega-3 fatty acids during pregnancy and lactation interferes with normal visual function and impairs learning ability in offspring, and may make the brain more susceptible to the damaging effects of environmental toxins and alcohol.

The Buzz on Omega-3s

Here's what medical experts are saying about the omega-3s:

Heart Disease and High Blood Pressure

- "The low incidence of coronary heart disease among Eskimos is related to their diet rich in marine fatty acids, which contain large amounts of polyunsaturated omega-3 fatty acids, mainly eicosapentaenoic and docosahexaenoic acids."[1]
- Dietary supplementation with fish oil delays the formation of blood clots that can cause heart attacks and strokes, probably by preventing blood cells from clumping and reducing damage to the arterial linings.[2]
- Dietary fish oil supplementation leads to reductions in blood pressure and triglycerides, and prevents blood clumping in people with obesity, high blood pressure and elevated blood lipids and cholesterol.[3]
- Smokers who cannot overcome their addiction should be encouraged "to use supplementary fish oil and other cardioprotective nutrients."[4]

High Cholesterol

- "Triglyceride lowering is the most consistent effect of fish oils."[5]
- Fish oil reduces total cholesterol and elevated beneficial high-density lipoproteins.[6]

Heart Attack Prevention

- The dietary intake of omega-3 fatty acids from seafood..."is associated with a reduced risk of primary cardiac arrest in humans."[7]
- The omega-3 fatty acid EPA is capable of salvaging the smooth muscle cells of the heart from post-heart attack damage.[8]
- "Fish oil...possibly due to the presence of n-3 fatty acids, may provide rapid protective effects in patients with acute myocardial infarction [heart attack]."[9]
- Early onset heart disease can be helped by "the multiple beneficial actions of n-3 fatty acids."[10]

Alzheimer's Disease

- Dietary fish oil/GLA "may slow or prevent Alzheimer's disease..."[11]

Pregnancy

- "Fish oil supplementation reduced the recurrence risk of pre-term delivery..."[12]

Autoimmunity

- The fish oil DHA inhibits an overactive immune system; thus, "DHA may be a useful agent in the treatment of conditions such as autoimmune disease."[13]

Rheumatoid arthritis

"Use of fish oil improved the number of tender joints and duration of morning stiffness at 3 months as analyzed by both meta- and meganalysis."[14]

"Patients taking dietary supplements of fish oil exhibit improvements in clinical parameters of disease activity from baseline, including the number of tender joints." These improvements are associated with significant decreases in levels of the pro-inflammatory chemical messenger interleukin-1 beta. "Some patients who take fish oil are able to discontinue NSAIDs (anti-inflammatory drugs) without experiencing a disease flare."[15]

Patients using fish oil supplements "were able to reduce their NSAID requirement without experiencing any deterioration in the clinical and laboratory parameters of RA activity."[16]

Psoriasis

According to several authors, fish oil is able not only to produce good clinical results, but also to minimize the side effects of retinoid therapy.[17]

Cancer

"Fish oil consumption is associated with protection against the promotional effects of animal fat in colorectal and breast carcinogenesis."[18]

Supplementing fish oils during the postoperative period "may reduce the number of infections and gastrointestinal complications per patient, as well as improve" kidney and liver function.[19]

"Hyperproliferation" (rapid cell division) is associated with an increased risk for colon cancer. A recent clinical trial found that fish-oil supplementation reduced the rate of proliferation in the upper crypt cells of patients with a history of colon polyps.[20]

The observation of a modification of the lipids of leukemia cells in a patient with chronic leukemia provides a biochemical basis for a possible beneficial effect of fish oil supplements on cancer-related wasting and tumor growth.[21]

Diabetes and Related Complications

The use of fish oil lowers triglyceride levels effectively by almost 30 percent. "Fish oil may be useful in treating dyslipidemia (elevated levels of tryglycerides) in diabetes."[22]

Treatment with a moderate daily dose of fish oil over a prolonged period of time significantly reduced triacylglycerol concentrations without any worsening of glucose tolerance in patients with high triglycerides and without impaired blood sugar levels.[23]

Kidney (Renal) Disease

Studies indicate protection against progressive renal disease after daily treatment for two years with fish oil providing 1.8 grams of eicosapentaenoic and 1.2 grams of docosahexaenoic acids.[24]

Continued on page 16...

...*Continued from page 15*

Peptic Ulcer

"*Helicobacter pylori* infection is currently treated with antimicrobial agents in combination with antacids. Recent studies have described the *in vitro* bactericidal activity of fish oils and polyunsaturated fatty acids on *H. pylori,* and reduced rates of duodenal ulcer in people with high intake of these substances...."[25]

Venereal Warts (Human Papilloma Virus)

"Docosahexaenoic acid inhibited growth of these [HPV-infected] cells to a greater extent than eicosapentaenoic acid. The effect of docosahexaenoic acid was dose dependent and caused growth arrest. Docosahexaenoic acid inhibited growth of HPV16 of the foreskin. Docosahexaenoic acid even inhibited growth in the presence of estradiol, a growth stimulator for these cells.[26]

Migraines

"Fish oil, owing to its platelet-stabilizing and antivasospastic actions, may also be useful in this regard, as suggested by a few clinical reports."[27,28]

IQ & Psychological Well Being

Dr. Barbara Levine, professor of nutrition in medicine at Cornell University, sounds the alarm concerning a totally inadequate intake of DHA by most Americans, according to a report summarized at the prestigious online International Health Database.[29] DHA is the building block of human brain tissue and is particularly abundant in the gray matter of the brain and the retina. Low levels of DHA have recently been associated with depression, memory loss, dementia, and visual problems. DHA is particularly important for fetuses and infants; the DHA content of the infant's brain triples during the first three months of life. Optimal levels of DHA are therefore crucial for pregnant and lactating mothers. Unfortunately, the average DHA content of breast milk in the United States is the lowest in the world, most likely because Americans eat comparatively little fish. Making matters worse is the fact that the United States is the only country in the world where infant formulas are not fortified with DHA. This despite a 1995 recommendation by the World Health Organization that all baby formulas should provide 40 milligrams (mg) of DHA per kilogram of infant body weight. Dr. Levine believes that postpartum depression, attention deficit hyperactivity disorder (ADHD), and low IQs are all linked to the dismally low DHA intake common in the United States. Dr. Levine also points out that low DHA levels have been linked to low brain serotonin levels, which are connected to an increased tendency to depression, suicide, and violence. DHA is abundant in marine phytoplankton and cold water fish, and nutritionists now recommend that people consume two to three servings of fish every week to maintain DHA levels. If this is not possible, Dr. Levine suggests supplementing with 100 mg per day of DHA.

These omega-3 fatty acids also benefit cardiovascular disease, hyperlipidemia (high cholesterol), hypertension (high blood pressure), prevention of myocardial infarction (heart attack), Alzheimer's disease, improved pregnancy outcome, nutritionally superior lactation, rheumatoid arthritis, psoriasis, cancer, diabetes mellitus, and many other conditions.

To be frank, we put almost every one of our patients on fish or flax oil capsules because we have to make the assumption that almost all are deficient in this vital nutrient. We don't want our patients to miss out on these important, essential nutrients that play such a vital role in reducing overall inflammation the body (perhaps the leading underlying cause of degenerative disease today).

THE IMPORTANCE OF CELL MEMBRANES

Political boundaries often represent lines of demarcation between distinctly different peoples, cultures, landmasses, and governing systems. In biological systems, well-defined boundaries are critical to optimal functioning.

Modern science accepts that water is an absolute prerequisite for all life, as we know it on Earth. Water is the dynamically active solvent that participates in all biochemical reactions that sustain life. But in order for life to express itself as individual life forms, water, and all of the biochemical activities it supports, must be compartmentalized into little packets of living substances. The boundaries that allow life to be so individuated are cell walls and membranes.

One of the structural features that distinguishes plants and animals is the fact that plant cells have walls made of carbohydrates, whereas animal cells have membranes made of fatty acids. Few people appreciate the fact that even the fatty acids on animal cell membranes have plant origins. Another distinguishing feature is plant storage of energy as carbohydrates (roots, tubers, etc.), while animals store energy as fat.

In animal cells, there are three major boundaries: the cell membrane, the nuclear membrane (surrounding the nucleus containing chromosomal DNA), and the mitochondrial membrane (surrounding the energy-producing organelles containing what are known as the mitochondrial DNA).

What is so important about membranes? As with political boundaries between nations, there are controls in place to restrict and influence what enters the cell, nucleus, and mitochondria, as well as what influence substances in contact with the membranes have on structures that reside within. Because of the far-reaching influence membranes have on cell functions, many cell biologists and other researchers even believe that a large number of diseases begin at the membrane level.

How well membranes perform depends on the quality of their structures. Fatty acids and cholesterol, held in place by water molecules, are the major structural components. Protein channels, spanning cell membranes, allow water-soluble substances to traverse the fatty components to enter the cell. Membrane surface proteins also serve as receptors for substances (for example, hormones or peptides) that will influence cell behavior.

When it comes to membrane fatty acids, what we eat is what we get. The fatty acids on the sperm and egg that joined to conceive the unique person that is you came from your parents' diets. The fatty acids on your cell membranes as you developed during pregnancy came from your mother's diet. The fatty acids you received from your mother in breast milk also came from her diet. From then on, the fatty acids in your diet became the fatty acids on your membranes. You became what you ate. (And if you aren't eating right, there is hope, because you can become what you eat and improve the health of your cellular membranes with omega-3s.)

Fatty acids are the building blocks for the three major membranes found in cells throughout the body—the outer cell membrane, the nuclear membrane, and the mitochondrial (cellular energy powerhouse) membrane. It is readily apparent from this wide dissemination of fatty acids why omega-3s have such a profound influence on cell function. A healthy diet, rich in omega-3 fatty acids, provides sufficient amounts of omega-3s to permeate the membranes of every single one of the body's one-hundred trillion cells. Our cell membranes should be composed mainly of the omega-3s. But, if they're not in the diet in adequate amounts, whatever is will be used. The functions of these membrane-supportive omega-3 fatty acids are of immense variety:

- serving as structural components of membranes;
- facilitating inter- and intra-cellular communication;
- regulating insulin production, as well as contributing to the manufacture of other endocrine hormones, thereby providing fatty acid raw materials for the manufacture of local tissue hormones—prostaglandins and leukotrienes—that influence blood pressure, inflammation, smooth muscle tonicity, and other functions;
- and, finally, influencing the response of cells to endocrine hormones, including insulin and the steroidal hormones from the adrenal glands and the gonads.

Thus, omega-3 fatty acids are key to a health-promoting, disease-preventing diet.

TYPES OF FATTY ACIDS

There are many types of distinct fatty acids found in nature (see Figure 1). Alpha-linolenic acid (a member of the omega-3 family) and linoleic acids (an omega-

FATTY ACIDS MADE SIMPLE
FIGURE 1

The Omega-6 Family	The Omega-3 Family
Linoleic Acid (LA)	**Alpha-Linolenic Acid (LNA)**
(Found in vegetable oil, seeds and nuts.)	(Found in green leafy vegetables, flax, flaxseed oil, canola oil, walnuts and Brazil nuts.)
Your body converts LA into:	Your body converts LNA into:
–	–
Gamma-Linolenic Acid (GLA)	**Eicosapentaenoic Acid (EPA)**
(GLA is also found in borage and primrose oil.)	(EPA is also found in fish oil.)
Your body converts GLA into:	Your body converts EPA into:
–	–
Arachidonic Acid (AA)	**Docosahexaenoic Acid (DHA)**
(AA is also found in meat.)	(DHA is also found in fish oil.)
The Omega-6 Family of Eicosanoids (i.e., hormone messengers)	**The Omega-3 Family of Eicosanoids (i.e., hormone (messengers)**

6) are considered essential because the body has enzyme systems that can convert these into the other members of their respective families. This means that it would be wise to have both of these fats or other members of both their families to support normal cellular functions. These fats are considered essential for another reason: they must be obtained from food because your body cannot synthesize them. What you eat is what your cells get—no more and no less.

Why are certain fatty acids essential? Essential fatty acids (EFAs) have several vital functions. First, they help to optimize metabolism, oxygen utilization, and energy production. Second, EFAs and their derivatives are components of membranes that surround each cell, nucleus, and mitochondrion. Lack of EFAs causes cells to have difficulty controlling the substances that enter and leave the intra-cellular environment. Third, EFAs are essential to maintaining healthy cholesterol and triglyceride levels. Fourth, they are indispensable to the normal development of the brain and nervous system in the fetus and young children. In fact, EFAs are important nutrients for the central nervous system throughout our lives and they help to maintain health and well-being (from a psychological perspective) as we age.

Finally, from EFAs tissues synthesize local hormone-like substances called prostaglandins and leukotrienes. As with the fatty acids from which they are made, prostaglandins and leukotrienes have major regulating functions throughout the body. They regulate arterial muscle tone, sodium excretion through the kidneys, platelet stickiness, inflammatory response, and immune function. Much research is currently being conducted on these compounds because of these important functions, especially inflammatory response.

Unfortunately, it is estimated that more than 60 percent of the North American population is deficient in the omega-3 EFAs and overindulging on foods that supply the body with an excess of the omega-6s, creating a severe physiological imbalance between these EFA families. The first obvious symptom when we consume too much omega-6 fatty acids is inflammation and pain. Your hips, joints, and legs ache and the pain you feel is frequently due to this inflammatory state caused by these fatty acids. The cause for most of us is our diet. We are simply consuming the wrong foods—excess amounts of red meat, vegetable cooking oils like peanut, safflower, soy and corn oil, or just about anything that is fried, baked, or processed. These foods are rich in pro-inflammatory omega-6 fatty acids.

Think of this incredible fact: one of the most dangerous foods is corn. (And you probably thought it was good for you!) Research from the United Kingdom shows that not only is corn one of the most dangerous foods for causing arthritis symptoms, it is also loaded with omega-6 fatty acids. Wheat products can also trigger inflammation.

Few people know that most men have early expressions of prostate cancer by the time they're in their twenties. The same is true for women and breast cancer. Scientists throughout the world are now saying that more and more of our most common disorders today are rooted in inflammation caused by this imbalance. Cancer, heart disease, diabetes, arthritis, Alzheimer's, stroke, lupus, and fibromyalgia can all be linked with an inflammatory state.

It all comes down to diet. The foods you consume determine your inflammatory levels. Your body converts omega-6 fatty acids to arachidonic acid. The body's COX-2 enzyme converts arachidonic acid to prostaglandin E2, which can inflame joints and lead to pain.

Unfortunately, we are not consuming enough of the best foods such as salmon and flax (rich in omega-3 fatty acids) or other foods like ginger, turmeric, and green tea that also inhibit the body's activity of proinflammatory compounds. For the last thirty to forty years, we have increasingly consumed more of the omega-6 fatty acids. Indeed, some health experts estimate we consume ten to twenty times more of the omega-6 than the omega-3 fatty acids. Even the most conscientious consumer who consumes these healthy foods still needs supplemental help.

We say unfortunate for very good reason: heart disease and cancer are pathological causes of approximately 73 percent of deaths involving degenerative disease in North America. And both of these diseases are linked to EFA malnutrition and imbalances and inflammation. It appears that fat and oil nutrition, which could delay or prevent some forms of heart disease and cancer, has been neglected far too long. This oversight is not so anymore. A great deal has been learned about the reasons for widespread essential fatty acid deficiencies and the problems caused by this deficiency. The major obstacle to beneficial change is the massive seed oil industry. In an effort to supply an increasing demand, an elaborate refining process was developed. As you may have already figured out, by the time the oil has been heated, degummed, bleached, deodorized and preserved with synthetic antioxidants, there is very little nutritional value left. Also, the wrong kinds of fats have been popularized—synthetic trans fatty acids found in margarine and those oils which although relatively shelf stable are naturally low in omega-3 fatty acids, such as corn and safflower oils.

THE SCOURGE OF MODIFIED FATS

The problem does not stop there. The EFAs in oil that have been subjected to the refining process function differently in the body than the EFAs found in fresh, unrefined oils. Refining alters the structure and shape of EFAs. Although they can still fit into the same metabolic pathways, they cannot carry out the same vital biochemical functions. These altered fats can occupy the same positions in cell membranes as normal fats, but the enzymes that attempt to metabolize them will be deactivated. Normal fatty acid metabolism will be obstructed. Not only is it difficult to get adequate amounts of unadulterated EFAs from our modern refined foods, but also any altered and refined oils we eat literally block the absorption and utilization of untampered fats we do ingest. We must eliminate both problems to receive the full benefits EFAs offer.

Good Fat vs. Bad Fat

So which are the good fats and which are the bad ones? A key to maintaining your body and mind in a state of optimum health is to learn to discern good fats from bad. In Greece and Italy, the typical diet consists of 40 percent fat (the same percentage as in the United States). But Greek and Italian men and women have significantly lower rates of prostate and breast cancer, as well as heart disease. This tells us that it isn't fat per se that is the enemy, but the type of fat. The Greek and Italian diet is loaded with omega-3 and monounsaturated olive oil (omega-9) fatty acids. These are the good fats that we don't get enough of from out diet anymore because our diet is laden with adulterated omega-6 fatty acids derived from refined vegetables oils such as corn and safflower, as well as hydrogenated oils (a source of dangerous trans-fatty acids) used to manufacture stick and tube margarine and as a baking ingredient.

Good fats can make quite a difference in your lifelong health. In combination with a consistent higher intake of organic vegetables, whole grains, and whole fruits, an adequate intake of beneficial omega-3 fats appears to be protective against breast cancer, observes researcher Emanuela Taioli. Similarly, low breast cancer rates in southern Italy are thought to be due to diets that avoid dangerous saturated fats. Interestingly, rates are higher in the north, where French cooking, rich in butterfat, predominates.[30] The diet in southern Italy also lacks the dangerous adulterated, human-made confection called margarine, a major source for trans-fatty acids. Researchers have found a high incidence of breast cancers in rodents fed a diet high in margarine.[31]

The Israeli Experience

Israel has dietary customs that include one of the highest intakes of polyunsaturated and saturated fats in the world. The consumption of omega-6 polyunsaturated fatty acids, found in safflower, corn and other highly processed commercial cooking oils, is about eight percent higher than in the United States and ten to twelve percent higher than in most European countries.

In fact, Israeli Jews may be regarded as a population-based dietary experiment exhibiting the effects of a high omega-6 and saturated fat diet. Not surprisingly, there is an extremely high prevalence of cardiovascular diseases, hypertension, non-insulin-dependent diabetes mellitus and obesity among Israeli Jews. There is also increased cancer incidence and mortality, especially in women, compared with Western countries. Studies suggest that high omega-6 fatty acid consumption might be the cause.[32]

Beyond Israel, the problem of consuming high amounts of bad fats at the expense of good fat appears to be of truly worldwide significance. Michael Murray, N.D., comments, "Most people have decreased their consumption of natural, unadulterated essential fatty acids and drastically increased their consumption of refined and adulterated fats and oils."

This trend is most unfortunate. Like Israelis, most of us need to get the undesirable fats out of our diet and incorporate more of the desirable ones.

Attack of the Killer Fats

You've heard about *"The Attack of the Killer Tomatoes,"* that goofy cult film. Well, imagine something far more insidious, killing you slowly without manifesting any clear adverse effects until you are stricken with a heart attack, stroke, or cancer. Dramatic scientific research shows that excess saturated fats and trans-fatty acids are such insidious creatures. Trans-fatty acids are so dangerous even the medical establishment is finally beginning to recognize the detrimental effects trans-fats have on the enzymes that metabolize fats. Major sources of trans-fatty acids are the hydrogenated vegetable oils used in margarine, vegetable shortening, baked goods, and many prepared foods. Another major source is the vegetable oils damaged by their continuous re-use in deep fat frying in restaurants, especially fast food, take-out and drive-through joints. These artificial fats increase risk for heart disease, cancer, diabetes, and other age-related maladies. Removing these obstacles to wellness will go a long way in improving your health.

Why You Need a Tablespoon of Omega-3-rich Oil Daily

Hippocrates, considered to be the father of medicine in Western civilization, advised people to let food be their medicine. This advice can easily be understood relative to fish oils. Both are rich in one of nature's most perfect fats to incorporate into your diet: omega-3 fatty acids.

Accumulating evidence from molecular and cellular biology, animal studies, and preliminary human clinical trials suggest that omega-3 fatty acids may potentially confer important health benefits related to reduced risk of cardiovascular disease, cancer, and diabetes, among other killer diseases today. These potential health benefits are consistent with epidemiological evidence that incidence of heart disease, various cancers, and menopausal symptoms are much lower among populations that consume plant-based diets rich in lignans and omega-3 fatty acids from flax or seafood.[33]

People of all ages can benefit from omega-3s. They are well on their way to becoming one of the most successful products in the health food industry due to their preventive and healing properties.

While removing the trans fats from your eating habits, consume wild ocean fish twice a week, such as wild salmon or tuna, and take omega-3-rich fish oils. The key is to both increase omega-3s and decrease omega-6s.

CHAPTER 2

Overfed and Undernourished–
Omega-3 Fatty Acid Deficiency
A Major Cause of Disease

Many nutritionists and natural health practitioners would agree that the American pop-ulation is overfed (in calories, refined carbohydrates, saturated fats, hydrogenated fats, and omega-6 oils) and undernourished (in pure water, vitamins, minerals, co-factors, and fiber). The eating habits of most people leave them in a state of essential fatty acid deficiency.

Imagine the impact of a shift in dietary patterns so rapid and radical that it adversely affects thousands of bodily metabolic functions simultaneously. Perhaps a worldwide famine, global pollution, and/or radiation could pose such a threat by contaminating or robbing our food of nutrients. Such a scenario is not merely hypothetical, but exists here and now. Though not as obvious as a global catastrophe, the true cause is much more insidious and began with the industrial revolution and the processing of foodstuffs to facilitate national and global transportation, packaging, and stability.

Throughout human history, men and women have ingested an approximate equal proportion (1:1) of omega-6 to omega-3 fatty acids. The omegas 6 and 3 are two of 49 known essential nutrients. As essential nutrients they cannot be synthesized by the body, but must be ingested directly in foods or in the form of dietary supplements.

The relationship of equivalence between the two omegas is critical because they self-check each other in a delicate balance to regulate thousands of metabolic functions through prostaglandin pathways.

Nearly every biologic function is somehow interconnected with the delicate balance between omega-6 and omega-3 fatty acids. As I mentioned, the omega-3s are intimately involved in the control of inflammation, cardiovascular health, myelin sheath develop-ment, allergic reactivity, immune response, hormone modulation, IQ, and behavior. A seemingly minor, yet major change in omega balance dictated by dietary ingestion has absolute deleterious health effects. The rapid change in dietary fat ingestion within only the last 50 to 100 years has bewildered human biophysiology created to function opti-mally on equal proportions of dietary omegas.

Diets that provide omega-6 oils at the expense of omega-3s stimulate pro-inflammatory pathways in the body, while omega-3s on the other hand stimulate anti-inflammatory pathways. As a result omega-6s have been coined as "bad" and omega-3s as "good." In fact, both are essential for human health and it is the balance of the two in relation to each other that is important. Dominant omega-6s in the body can create a situation that promotes chronic inflammation, cancer, heart disease, stroke, diabetes, arthritis and auto-immunity.

THE INDUSTRIAL REVOLUTION & SEED OILS

It has long been known that, unless heroic preservation measures are taken, once flaxseed and other seed grains are crushed that they soon turn rancid. Because of the high vulnerability of their electrons to oxidation, these precious oils, much like fruits or vegetables, are highly perishable. The husks and germs of grains first began to be removed in the mid-1700s in Great Britain, extending shelf life but removing their vital contents, thereby precipitating overt B-vitamin deficiency diseases such as pellagra and beriberi. The vital powers of these seed-rich foods were lost. Then along came the corn oil craze in the 1950s. The producers of the commodity launched a massive public misinformation campaign, taking out full-page advertisements in the nation's medical journals. This campaign convinced medical doctors that corn oil, so overloaded with omega-6 fatty acids, could prevent heart disease.

Most people don't realize that many of the vegetable oils we take for granted today were only introduced into common usage in recent years, since the Industrial Revolution. The development of screw-nut expeller presses allowed the mass extraction of oil from seeds and nuts not commonly used by large populations of people—corn, safflower, sunflower. These are the vegetable oils rich in omega-6 and devoid of omega-3 fatty acids. As industrialization permeated all aspects of mass food production, the processing of food for maximum shelf life, rather than nutritional value, became the number one goal. Foods rich in omega-3 fatty acids began to be excluded because they have a shorter shelf life than those with omega-6 fatty acids and hydrogenated fats. Thus, the manufacturers and retailers of processed foods deliberately excluded sources of omega-3 fats in order to maximize marketability.

MODERN ANIMAL HUSBANDRY

The herbivorous animals domesticated as livestock for human consumption were designed by their Creator and Nature to eat green vegetation, the principal food available to them in the wild, not the grains upon which livestock are commonly raised. In fact, virtually all herbivores in the wild live on green leaves, not the seeds. The practitioners of modern animal husbandry, in contrast to the way Nature nourishes herbivores, have chosen to rely on grain as a major food source for certain reasons. Livestock raised on grain grow faster, fatter, and cheaper. Unfortunately, their tissue is high in omega-6 fatty acids, in contrast to range-fed animals and wild game that are rich in omega-3. Eggs, once a good source of omega-3s, have also fallen victim to progress. Chickens, like cattle, are fed a diet absent of omega-3s, and as a result their eggs are also deficient. Fish, perhaps the most well known source of omega-3, have also been negatively effected. Chances are, the fish on your dining table was "farm raised" and did not eat phytoplankton that creates omega-3s. That's why we think a quality omega-3 supplement from pollution-free ocean sources is vital to your health. (Also, seek DHA-enriched eggs, now widely available in supermarkets.)

HYDROGENATION

As previously mentioned, refined food manufacturers were quick to learn that omega-3s significantly decreased the shelf life and therefore the marketability of their products. Dietary sources of omega-3 were and continue to be purposely avoided in the production of processed foods. Another wrong turn was the use of compounds in hydrogenation, a process that turns vegetable oils into semi-solid fats. The beauty of the omega-3 fatty acids is that they won't solidify at room temperature. You can freeze omega-3-rich oil and it won't solidify. Thus it remains fluid in cell membranes (no wonder it's so good for rheumatism!).

When most Americans see on the label of a processed food or vegetable shortening the phrase "hydrogenated vegetable oil," they really don't understand what that phrase means or its undesirable health implications. Vegetable oils, usually high in polyunsaturated fatty acids, are liquid at room temperature. In order to produce a vegetable shortening that can stay semi-solid at room temperature, vegetable oil must be partially hydrogenated. To add hydrogen to the unsaturated bonds of vegetable fatty acids, manufacturers heat the oil in the presence of a catalyst (for example, nickel) and bubble hydrogen through the mixture. The result is a man-made "plastic" used to give processed foods a particular texture and desired "mouth feel" that American palates have been cultivated to find desirable.

Yet this kind of artificial chemical manipulation of vegetable oils induces undesirable long-term consequences. In their zeal to avoid health problems linked to ingestion of saturated animal fats, people inadvertently ran into other health difficulties. For example, it is intriguing that after the masses abandoned butter and lard for margarine, vegetable shortening, and omega-6 cooking oils, the risk of vascular disease went down while the risk of cancer went up.

EXPORTING WESTERN ILLNESSES TO ASIA

In a landmark study, Japanese researchers have discovered this EFA imbalance to be a leading cause for the advent of Western degenerative diseases in Japan. We now have strong evidence that omega-3 fatty acid deficiency could be one of the most important risk factors for the most deadly, disabling diseases of modern times.

Researchers noticing the proliferation of Western degenerative diseases among Japanese natives asked what had changed in their diet or way of life. Why, they asked, are the people of Japan—who once seemed almost impervious to typical Western maladies and whose life expectancy is markedly greater than that of Americans—suddenly suffering many of the same diseases as other inhabitants of industrialized nations?

The answers have come from Japanese researchers, whose recent published work appears to confirm a mountain of emerging scientific discoveries stating that the lack of omega-3 fatty acids in the modern Japanese diet is a major cause of degenerative diseases. Skyrocketing ingestion of omega-6 fatty acids compounds the problem.

In the West, we may love our sunflower, safflower, peanut, and corn oils, but these are replete in omega-6 fatty acids, and devoid of beneficial omega-3s. These omega-6 vegetable oils are being consumed far more frequently in Japan than ever before, as the American diet begins to permeate the Japanese culture. The results are clear: the Japanese people, more than ever, are becoming susceptible to our Western diseases.

"Western" is an appropriate adjective because Western industrial societies that consume their uniquely refined diets have a much higher incidence of these diseases, compared to peoples consuming unrefined indigenous diets. These maladies include

FYI: Inflammatory Diseases You Can Prevent or Heal with More Omega-3 Fatty Acids in your Diet

We now know that an undesirable tendency toward chronic inflammation is at the heart of many of our most common and debilitating chronic diseases. But fish oils can help significantly. Inflammation-related diseases that you can prevent or for which you can induce healing with the omega-3 fatty acids in wild ocean fish include heart disease, rheumatoid arthritis, lupus, and even cancer. There is now some evidence that chronic inflammation predisposes persons to increased risk for Alzheimer's disease. Thus, a diet rich in omega-3 fatty acids may prevent each of these conditions.

Because omega-3 fatty acids are so quickly assimilated into the body and often in short supply, their effects can be quite rapid. Within days of putting them into your diet, your body's inflammatory condition will begin to respond.

This can be confirmed with a high-sensitivity C-reactive protein test, used to monitor inflammatory conditions. (Your doctor can do this test. The cost is only about $50 and usually covered by insurance.)

heart disease, cancer, stroke, diabetes, arthritis, obesity, and chronic immune deficiency. Tragically, the American diet is the most refined of all. To make matters worse, this Standard American Diet (whose acronym ironically is SAD) is being disseminated all over the world with serious pathological consequences.

OMEGA-3 FATTY ACIDS: 'ESSENTIAL' FOR HEALTH AND LIFE

Why do Western diseases bear a striking association with a lack of dietary omega-3 fatty acids? Omega-3 fatty acids are indispensable cellular building blocks. These nutrients must be ingested as food or nutritional supplementation. There are no enzymes in the human body that can convert other classes of fatty acids (omega-6 or omega-9) into omega-3 fats. If you don't eat omega-3s, you don't get omega-3s. Each of our 100 trillion cells should be supplied with an optimal amount of omega-3 fatty acids. Within the cell wall, omega-3 fatty acids serve to secure structural integrity, as well as facilitate cellular respiration.

In the absence of adequate omega-3 fatty acids, the body must use less desirable fatty acids as surrogates (omega-6 fatty acids and even saturated fats), leading to compromised cellular integrity and overall health.

In particular, without our omega-3 fatty acids, the body goes into a state of chronic inflammation. The body's inflammatory response is beneficially influenced by omega-3 fatty acids. The inflammatory response was created or evolved as a healing reaction to acute injury or microbial attack. However, if the inflammatory response is needlessly provoked or prolonged, unnecessary damage will occur to tissues and organs of the body. The omission of adequate omega-3 fatty acids in the diets of people among the industrialized nations has created a tendency toward chronic inflammation among many people. In this case, symptoms of inflammation precede the full expression of diseases such as circulatory problems and cancer. However, as unbridled inflammation tends to perpetuate itself, leading to chronic disease, a vicious circle of inflammation and disease is formed.

The "essentiality" of omega-3 fatty acids cannot be denied. In fact, a deficiency of omega-3 fatty acids in the diet can be considered as a reliable indicator or predictor of the risk of disease. Given the research that indicates most individuals are deficient in omega-3 fatty acids, it can be accurately stated that the majority of these individuals will suffer compromised health or premature death as a result.

Making matters worse for the Japanese population is the importation of American dietary habits. This has led to mass consumption of undesirable omega-6 fatty acids, found in high concentrations in common vegetable oils and foods made from such oils. These are the kinds of oils people are eating more and more frequently throughout the nation; thanks to the dissemination of American fast food exports, these unhealthy foods are being inflicted upon the entire human population of the *world*. The massive ingestion of omega-6 fatty acids, out of proportion to omega-3 fatty acids, wreaks havoc on the body's metabolism and inherent protection against deadly diseases.

Put bluntly: American dietary habits exported abroad are killing the Japanese.

Japanese researchers have documented this dietary shift toward omega-6 fatty acids at the expense of omega-3s. Currently, the Japanese ingest four times as much omega-6 as they do omega-3 fatty acids. This trend is bad enough, but not nearly as troubling as in the United States, where people consume an average of *twenty times* more omega-6 fatty acids than omega-3 fatty acids! Unfortunately, trends in Japan indicate that nation's population may soon match the omega-6 fatty acid intake of Americans.

"Most researchers describe a healthy balance of omega-6 to omega-3 oils as anywhere from 1:1, to 3 or 4:1," notes nutritionist Lalitha Davis, author of *10 Essential Foods* (Hohm Press, 1997). "You probably won't be surprised to learn that the balance of these two essential fatty acids in the body of the average American is about 20:1! This basic nutrient imbalance (way more omega-6 than is healthy in balance with omega-3) is caused by a diet high in processed and refined foods, grocery store vegetable oils which are highly refined with toxic chemicals, and domestic animal meats."

The commercial extraction of seed oils dominant in omega-6 fatty acids and their widespread use in prepared foods has resulted in an extremely high intake of omega-6 fatty acids in the diet (see Figure 2). Before the

Figure 2

Fueling the Fire

Foods, vegetable oils and nutritional supplements dominant in, or equal in proportion of Omega-3 to Omega-6 fatty acids.

	Omega-6	Omega-3	Ratio
Processed Foods	varies	None	100/0
Safflower Oi	79%	None	100/0
Sunflower Oil	69%	None	100/0
Corn Oil	60%	None	100/0
Peanut	30%	None	100/0
Walnut	51%	5%	5/1
Soy Oil	50%	8%	6/1
Canola Oil	24%	10%	2.5/1

Industrial Revolution, people consumed an appropriate one-to-one ratio of omega-6 to omega-3 fatty acids in grains and green foods, and from the tissues of livestock animals and hunted game. The animals consumed then were also rich in omega-3 fats because they were feeding on green vegetation, the original source of omega-3 fatty acids.

Now, consider the typical fast food meal or prepared convenience foods: French fries, salad dressing, hamburgers and other fried meats are loaded with omega-6 fatty acids and almost devoid of omega-3 fatty acids. And to make matters even more disturbing, the same oil, loaded with trans fatty acids, is used to deep fry potatoes, onion rings, chicken, and other favorites, and it has been reused day after day for up to three months, when the franchise management finally allows the oil in the deep fat fryer to be changed. The oxidative and other molecular damage done to these already questionable oils is absolutely horrendous—and the same highly reactive molecules in the oil are dumped into our bodies! The oil is laden with rancid, oxidized fats, which generate free radicals, toxic molecules that attack our cellular genetic material and are thought to be the underlying cause of molecular changes leading to the aging process, cancer, heart disease, cataracts, and many other of our most common conditions. And people are daily gobbling food cooked in this waste by the ton. Is there any wonder why we have chronic health problems?

MONUMENTAL RESEARCH

There has been growing concern by Japanese government and public health officials, as well as a growing legion of health professionals, who have noted a correlation between the adoption of an Americanized diet and a drastic rise in death and disability attributed to degenerative disease. In addition to debilitating illness, the number of allergy patients has increased several-fold in the past 40 years. Today in Japan, one of every three Japanese infants born is diagnosed as allergy-hyperreactive.

It was this concern that motivated Japanese researchers at Nagoya City University, Faculty of Pharmaceutical Sciences, to investigate the causes of the rise of Western degenerative disease in Japan. The results of their research have been published in the prominent medical journal *Progress in Lipid Research,* occupying 50 pages.

An intensive research study was undertaken which included a thorough review of nearly 500 existing studies related to the issue.

One such review was that of the drastic decline in the health of the people of Okinawa since the advent of American presence on that island.

THE OKINAWA EXPERIENCE

Citizens of the prefecture of Okinawa used to hold the unique distinction of having the highest longevity among the 47 prefectures of Japan, and, indeed, the world. However, Okinawa was under the jurisdiction of the U.S. following World War II, up until 1972. The Western habitation of the islands began to negatively influence the traditional diet by dramatically increasing consumption of omega-6 dominant vegetable oils. The magnitude of this change was such that by 1975 the amount of vegetable oil purchased per household was two-fold higher in Okinawa than in other parts of Japan. The lifestyle of the Okinawan people also shifted from a diet whose major animal protein source was fish, rich in omega-3 fatty acids, to meat. The combination of a diet high in vegetable oil and low in fish created a drastic shift in the omega-6 to omega-3 fatty acid ratio. Consequently, there was a corresponding rise in degenerative disease. Sadly, the rest of Japan has reached or surpassed Okinawa in consumption of omega-6 dominant oils, as well as the processed and baked foods that contain them.

By 1990, the longevity of Okinawan males was fifth among Japanese prefectures, which was a drastic decline from the previous top position. The recent trends in lipid nutrition and disease patterns in Okinawa are thus characterized by the most rapid Westernization among the Japanese prefectures. Although the Westernization of cooking and eating habits in Okinawa has preceded the rest of Japan, the other regions have quickly gained ground.

Unfortunately, the Japanese people engaged in these changes failed to realize that they were unwittingly enlisted in a race to an early grave. It is an accurate statement, say these researchers, that the most predictive factor for a shortened life span in Japan, if not the world, is a deficiency of omega-3 fatty acids in the diet, relative to omega-6 fatty acids. The retrospective analysis of the Okinawan diet simply serves as a microcosmic insight into the imbalances in the American diet, which caused Americans to suffer the same fate nearly 60 years earlier.

Perhaps equally as important as the preventative qualities of omega-3 fatty acids are their curative ones. The Japanese researchers found that an omega-3 fatty acid-rich diet, derived from vegetable sources, is helpful in healing breast, colon, rectal and kidney tumors. These findings became even more apparent as the percentage of omega-6 was reduced.

CHILDHOOD BEHAVIORAL DISORDERS IN JAPAN ARE ON THE RISE

The Japanese have long been lauded for their high intellect and impeccably controlled decorum. However, today in Japan they are faced with escalating incidences of attention deficit disorder and other behavior and learning problems. The traditional Japanese diet, high in omega-3 fatty acids, may have been a contributing factor to the behavioral health and intellectual vitality of these people. It is believed by researchers that eighty percent of the lipids in the cerebral cortex of the brain should be composed of omega-3 fatty acids, with 35 percent in the form of docosahexaenoic acid (DHA). For many Japanese children, this severe deficiency has lowered the omega-3 fatty acid concentrations found in brain tissue. These children are more likely to suffer from hyperactivity and similar behavioral disorders.

OMEGA-3S FOR VIBRANT HEALTH AND LONGEVITY

According to Artemis Simopoulos, M.D., president of the Center for Genetics, Nutrition and Health, it would take the human body more than one-million years to adapt the radical change in ingestion of omega-6 to omega-3 fatty acids that has occurred only within the last 100 years in America and in the last 50 years for the Japanese.

In other words, this is not a problem that is going to go away on its own. The implications are clear. We must ingest omega-3 fats in our diets and in supplements to avert otherwise certain degenerative diseases.

Positive changes are occurring in health food stores across America and through-out the world, as consumers are flocking to one of the hottest products on the mar-ket—omega-3s. A recent nationwide survey in the United States put awareness of omega-3 on par with antioxidants, revealing a 54 percent awareness level among adult consumers.

Likewise, savvy Japanese citizens are utilizing flaxseed oil as a dressing to their tradi-tional morning salad. Incorporating flax oil into a staple, such as the morning salad, is a method that could positively impact lives of countless multitudes of Japanese.

The ingestion of fresh, wild deepwater fish and toxin-free fish oil supplements also raises the body's omega-3 stores. Consuming the right seafood is extremely important.

OPTIMAL HEALTH IN THE BALANCE

The ratio of fatty acids in the diet goes a long way in determining risk for many dis-eases. The difference in proportions between the American and Japanese populations helps to explain why the Japanese, until just recently, have not manifested many of the "degenerative" Western diseases. The ratio of omega-6 to omega-3 fatty acids in the typ-ical US diet is 10:1 to 20:1. But the ratio has been 4:1 in Japan until the recent deluge of American fast junk food. Now the Japanese are eating the kinds of fats Americans do and are suffering the consequences to their health.

The consumption of omega-6 in North America represents seven percent of caloric intake (about 15 grams daily). The consumption of omega-3 in this population is 0.0 to 0.3 percent of calories. Amazingly, people in the upper quintile of that low range for omega-3s (0.66 grams daily) have 40 percent fewer cardiovascular deaths. So even slight improvements can provide significant benefits.

How can we correct this tremendous imbalance? Decrease the intake of omega-6 fatty acid sources. This includes omega-6 vegetable oils, hydrogenated oils, processed foods, products from grain-raised livestock, and farmed fish. Prefer products from range-fed livestock, wild ocean fish, fish oil, and walnut and flax oils. For cooking, use olive oil, which has demonstrated its own health benefits, especially among Italians who have lower cardiovascular risk despite high olive oil consumption.

Perhaps most enlightening are the words of the Japanese researchers excerpted from the study summary:

> In this review, we summarize the evidence, which indicates that increased
> dietary linoleic acid (omega-6) and relative omega-3 deficiency are major risk
> factors for Western-type cancers cardiovascular and cerebrovascular diseases

and also for allergic hyper-reactivity. We also raise the possibility that a relative omega-3 deficiency may be affecting the behavioral patterns of a proportion of the young generations in industrialized countries.... It is proposed that dietary intervention with omega-3 fatty acids, and the reduction of omega-6 fatty acids in the diet, could successfully reverse the rising trend toward Westernized degenerative diseases in Japan, and the world.

Part II–
Omega-3s &
Your Health

Omega-3s for a Healthy Heart

Heart disease and its complications are the major causes of death in the United States and have reached epidemic proportions throughout the Western world. "Heart disease" is a term that is used commonly to describe atherosclerotic disease of the coronary arteries. Heart attacks, strokes, and other cardiovascular events related to atherosclerosis (hardening of the arteries), blood clotting, and vascular spasm are responsible for roughly 43 percent of all deaths in the United States.

Now we have good evidence that fish oil supplements might just save your life. This is not our opinion but the opinion expressed in the May 27, 2003 issue of the highly prestigious American Heart Association journal *Circulation*. In a landmark editorial clinicians advocate, "There is a need to consider a new indication for treatment with low-dose n-3 PUFA [omega-3 fatty acid or fish oil] supplements—the prevention of sudden cardiac death in patients with a prior [heart attack]."

The *Circulation* editorial continues to say that eating wild oily fish like salmon, sardines, or mackerel at least twice a week can prevent sudden cardiac death because fatty acids in the fish block dangerous irregular heart rhythms. Of course, we've been telling patients to consume wild salmon, herring, sardines, trout and other fish rich in omega-3 fatty acids for some time. We've also advocated use of high-quality, laboratory-certified fish oil supplements due to pollution concerns with many species of popular fish (especially bluefish), and because altogether too many people simply won't consume adequate amounts of seafood. Also, some seafood favorites, such as salmon, are often farm-raised and suspected of providing limited amounts of valuable omega-3 fatty acids compared to their wild counterparts (due to differences in diets of farm-raised fish).

Researchers at the Veterans Affairs Medical Center report that DHA provides significant protection against the development of coronary heart disease.[35] Their study involved over 6,000 middle-aged men who had samples of their blood taken between 1973 and 1976. The researchers found that men with a higher blood level of the omega-3 unsaturated fatty acids had an almost 50 percent lower risk of developing heart disease than did men with lower levels. The researchers also found that men with CHD tended to have a higher serum level of omega-6 fatty acids derived from linoleic acid, but were unable to confirm previous reports that these acids are linked to an increased risk of CHD.

HOW FISH OILS PREVENT ARRHYTHMIAS

Epidemiologists have known for years that eating fish was associated with reduced risk of cardiovascular disease, but only recently have researchers had laboratory evidence to explain this effect, says lead author Alexander Leaf, M.D., Jackson Professor of Clinical Medicine Emeritus at Harvard Medical School in Boston. Leaf and his colleagues present a detailed explanation of how omega-3 (n-3) fish oils benefit the heart.

Animal experiments show that fatty acids from n-3 fish oils are stored in the cell membranes of heart cells and can prevent sudden cardiac death from fatal arrhythmias, which are irregular heart rhythms. Arrhythmias, especially those of the ventricles of the heart, are considered to be major contributing events in sudden cardiac death. Leaf says studies of individual heart cells demonstrate omega-3 fatty acids (n-3 PUFAs) specifically block excessive sodium and calcium currents in the heart. Those excessive electrical discharges cause dangerous and erratic changes in heart rhythm.

The first clinical suggestion that omega-3 fatty acids significantly benefit the heart came from a 1989 study in which 2,033 men with heart disease were given dietary advice on fat, fiber or fish. After two years the men who were told to eat fish at least twice a week had a 29 percent reduction in death. There was no benefit in either the fiber or fat groups.

Since about 50 to 60 percent of deaths from coronary heart disease are sudden cardiac deaths within one hour of symptoms, and are often attributed to sustained arrhythmias, the authors note the reduction in deaths reported in this early study was probably evidence of fewer fatal arrhythmias.

This initial study was followed by a series of observational studies and controlled clinical trials. All arrived at the same conclusion: a diet rich in fatty fish reduced fatal heart attacks. But this "protection" was still not completely understood.

In early animal experiments, researchers demonstrated that animals fed a diet in which 12 percent of the calories came from saturated fat died of sustained ventricular fibrillation, but animals that were also fed omega-3 fatty acids did not develop these dangerous arrhythmias when their coronary arteries were tied off. But then Leaf and other researchers still needed to find out if "there were any plausible biochemical or physiological effects of these n-3 fatty acids which could explain their antiarrhythmic action." To do so, they cultured neonatal heart cells from rats and observed them under the microscope. The cells clump together and the clump beats spontaneously, rhythmically and simultaneously just like the whole heart. Using a video camera, Leaf and his colleagues taped the action of the cells and the effect of different toxic agents on the cells. They discovered that adding the omega-3 fatty acids prevented arrhythmias induced in the cells.

The Beneficial Effects of Omega-3 Fatty Acids
on Cardiovascular Ailments

We also know that several large clinical trials have confirmed the ability of fish oils to prevent sudden cardiac death in both presumably healthy subjects as well as in patients having suffered a heart attack (myocardial infarction).[36] According to the International Health News Database, "Considering that sudden cardiac death, largely caused by ventricular fibrillation, accounts for somewhere between 250,000 and 300,000 deaths every year in the United States alone, it is clearly highly significant that a diet rich in oily fish or fish oil supplements may reduce the incidence of sudden cardiac death by up to 45 percent."

Recently published studies are clearly showing how protective omega-3 oils can be. An Italian study published in the April 2002 edition of *Circulation* involved more than 11,000 recent heart attacks patient randomly assigned to receive, in addition to their pharmaceutical medicines, omega-3 oils, vitamin E, both, or no additional treatment. Within three months of treatment, it became clear to researchers that omega-3s were significantly decreasing mortality risk. Within four months, the relative risk of sudden death in the omega-3 group was less than half that the untreated group. Within six to eight months, similar risk reduction was noted for cardiovascular, cardiac, and coronary deaths. What make these results even more impressive is that the dosage of omega-3s was only one gram daily. The research team concluded that the early effect of low-dose omega-3 fatty acids on total mortality and sudden death supports the hypothesis of an anti-arrhythmic effect.[37]

An American study published in the April 11, 2002 issue of *The New England Journal of Medicine* followed apparently healthy men over a period up to 17 years as part of the Physicians' Health Study. The fatty-acid composition of blood previously collected from 94 men in whom sudden death occurred as the first manifestation of cardiovascular disease was matched to 184 controls according to age and smoking status. Interestingly, base-line blood levels of omega-3 fatty acids were inversely related to the risk of sudden death. The relative risk of sudden death was dramatically lower among men with higher levels of omega-3s in their blood. The research group concluded that "the n-3 fatty acids found in fish are strongly associated with a reduced risk of sudden death among men without evidence of prior cardiovascular disease."[38]

The praise from many health professionals is overwhelming. According to health researcher Hans R. Hansen, M.Sc. Ch.E., "An enormous amount of medical literature testifies to the fact that fish oils... help maintain the elasticity of artery walls, prevent blood clotting, reduce blood pressure and stabilize heart rhythm."[39,40,41,42,43,44,45,46] Testimonies from other sources include Danish researchers concluding that fish oils may help prevent arrhythmias and sudden cardiac death in healthy men, a group of German researchers finding that fish oil supplementation for 2 years reduced atherosclerotic deposits, and American medical researchers reporting that men who consume fish once or more every week have a 50 percent lower risk of dying from a sudden cardiac event than do men who eat fish less than once a month.[47,48,49,50,51,52] Greek researchers report that ten grams of fish oil a day reduces the number of attacks in male angina sufferers by 41 percent. In Norway, medical doctors have found that fish oil supplementation reduces the severity of a heart attack. Indian researchers discovered that fish oil taken immediately after a heart attack reduces future complications.

Bypass surgery and angioplasty patients reportedly also benefit from fish oils; clinical trials have shown that they are safe for heart disease patients. An adequate daily intake (about 1 gram) of EPA and DHA is essential to maintain a healthy heart. Fish oils are especially important for diabetics who have an increased risk of heart disease.

Meanwhile, fish consumption lowers the heart rate. An elevated heart rate is associated with an increased risk of sudden cardiac death, says Larsen, who cites the example of the Paris Prospective Study that included more than 7,700 men observed over 23 years. According to the study, the average difference between controls and patients who died suddenly from cardiac arrest was 4.1 beats per minute (bpm). A group of European researchers now reports that regular fish consumption can lower heart rates by as much as two bpm. Their study included 9,758 men aged 50 to 59 years from Belfast, Lille, Strasbourg, and Toulouse. 27 percent of the men consumed fish less than once per week, 47 percent consumed fish once a week, 20 percent twice a week, and the remaining 6 percent more than twice a week. The average heart rate (adjusted for age, physical activity, smoking, alcohol consumption, etc.) was 67.5 bpm in men consuming fish less than once per week and 65.6 bpm in men consuming fish more than twice per week.

Fish consumers also had lower triglyceride levels, lower blood pressure (both systolic and diastolic), and higher levels of beneficial HDL cholesterol than did nonconsumers. The erythrocyte content of DHA (docosahexaenoic acid) in the blood was inversely correlated with the heart rate. The researchers point out considerable evidence that omega-3 fatty acids such as those found in fish and fish oils stabilize the electrical activity of heart cells. There is also evidence that a high omega-3 content of blood cells and serum cholesterol esters is associated with increased heart rate variability. A higher heart rate variability has been associated with a decreased risk of cardiac disease and a longer lifespan.[53]

FISH OIL & HIGH BLOOD PRESSURE (HYPERTENSION)

Hypertension is the medical term for high blood pressure, a condition with many causes. Approximately 90 percent of people with high blood pressure have "essential" or "idiopathic" hypertension, for which the cause is poorly understood. The terms "hypertension" and "high blood pressure" as used here refer only to this most common form and not to high blood pressure either associated with pregnancy or clearly linked to a known cause, such as Cushing's syndrome, adrenal tumors, or kidney disease.

Researchers at the University of Cincinnati have found that supplementing with as little as 2 grams/day of fish oil (410 mg of EPA plus 285 mg of DHA) can lower diastolic pressure by 4.4 mm Hg and systolic pressure by 6.5 mm Hg. This is enough to avoid taking drugs in cases of borderline hypertension. Several other clinical trials have confirmed that fish oils are indeed effective in lowering high blood pressure and that they may work even better if combined with a program of salt restriction.[54]

This is not to say that fish oil is by itself a guaranteed cure. As with conventional drugs, the use of natural substances sometimes controls blood pressure if taken consistently but does not mean a cure for high blood pressure. Hypertension must always be evaluated by a healthcare professional. Extremely high blood pressure (malignant hypertension) or rapidly worsening blood pressure (accelerated hypertension) almost always requires treatment with conventional medicine. People with mild to moderate high blood pressure should work with a doctor before attempting to use the information contained here, as blood pressure requires monitoring and, in some cases, the use of blood pressure-lowering drugs. Permanent changes in one's dietary habits, such as an increased intake of fruits and vegetables and less usage of salt, and regular exercise are necessary in order to maintain control of blood pressure.

HOLD THE SALT AND PASS THE SALAD, PLEASE—LESS COFFEE AS WELL

Eliminating salt from one's diet is quite difficult to achieve; with the prevalence of salted, processed, and restaurant food, simply avoiding the salt shaker no longer leads to large decreases in salt intake for most people. However, an overview of the best studies find that the more salt is restricted, the lower blood pressure levels become. Although individual studies sometimes come to differing conclusions about the relationship between salt intake and blood pressure—in part because the effects of salt restriction vary from person to person, and small to moderate reductions in salt intake often have minimal effects on blood pressure—dramatic reductions in salt intake are generally effective for many hypertensive people.

Another option is a vegetarian diet, which has been reported to significantly lower blood pressure. This occurs partly because fruits and vegetables contain potassium, a known blood pressure-lowering mineral. The best way to supplement potassium is with fruit, which contains more of the mineral than the amounts found in potassium supplements. However, fruit contains so much potassium that people taking "potassium-sparing" diuretics (as some hypertensives do) can end up with too much potassium by eating several pieces a day. Therefore, people using diuretics should consult the prescribing doctor before increasing their fruit intake.

The fiber provided by vegetarian diets may also help reduce high blood pressure. In the Dietary Approaches to Stop Hypertension (DASH) trial, increasing the intake of fruits and vegetables (and therefore fiber) and reducing cholesterol and dairy fat led to large reductions in blood pressure (in medical terms, 11.4 systolic and 5.5 diastolic) in just eight weeks.[55] Even though it did not employ a vegetarian diet itself, the outcome of the DASH trial supports the usefulness of vegetarian diets because diets employed by DASH researchers were related to what many vegetarians eat. The DASH trial also showed that blood pressure can be significantly reduced in hypertensive people (most dramatically in African Americans) with diet alone without weight loss or even restriction of salt.[56]

On the other hand, sugar and caffeine consumption has been reported to increase blood pressure. Though the real importance of this experimental effect remains somewhat unclear, some doctors recommend that people with high blood pressure cut back on their sugar intake.[57]

In an analysis of 11 trials lasting almost two months on average, coffee drinking led to increased blood pressure, though these increases were typically small to moderate.

LIFESTYLE CHANGES—REPLACING VICES WITH VIRTUOUS ACTIVITIES

Toss your Malboros away and pour your vodka down the drain. Smoking is particularly injurious, and unnecessary, for people with hypertension. The combination of hypertension and smoking greatly increases the risk of heart disease-related sickness and death. With respect to alcohol, many studies have found a relationship between its consumption and blood pressure; recent reports show that above the equivalent of approximately three drinks per day, blood pressure increases in proportion to the amount of alcohol consumed.[58]

Daily exercise can lower blood pressure significantly. People over 40 years of age should consult with their doctor before starting an exercise regime. A 12-week program of Chinese T'ai Chi was reported to be almost as effective as aerobic exercise in lowering blood pressure in sedentary elderly people with high blood pressure.

Many people with high blood pressure are overweight. Weight loss can lower blood pressure significantly in those who are both overweight and hypertensive. People with hypertension who are overweight should talk with a doctor about a weight loss program.[59]

Some nutritional supplements may be helpful, although their beneficial effects vary depending on the severity of one's hypertension. Calcium supplementation—typically 800 to 1,500 mg per day—lowers blood pressure. However, while an analysis of 42 trials reported that calcium supplementation led to an average drop in blood pressure that was *statistically* significant, the decrease was not large enough to meaningfully improve health (in medical terms, a drop of 1.4 systolic over 0.8 diastolic pressure).[60] Results would likely be better were analysis limited only to studies of hypertensive people, because calcium has little if any effect on those with normal blood pressure. Although average decreases in blood pressure from calcium are clearly small, each person responds differently. Some evidence suggests that people with hypertension whose blood pressure is affected most by changes in salt intake respond best to calcium supplementation.[61] A 12-week trial of 1,000 mg per day of calcium accompanied by blood pressure monitoring is a reasonable way to assess efficacy in a given individual.

In addition to calcium, some studies show that magnesium supplements—typically 350 to 500 mg per day—lower blood pressure.[62,63] Magnesium appears to be particularly effective in people who are taking potassium-depleting diuretics; because these diuretics also deplete magnesium, magnesium supplements may be credited with helping overcome a mild deficiency, leading to a drop in blood pressure.

Next, Vitamin C plays an important role in maintaining the health of arteries. A review of vitamin C research reported that most studies linked increased blood and dietary levels of the vitamin to reduced blood pressure. However, these links might result from diets high in fruits and vegetables, rather than from vitamin C itself. The same review reported that blood pressure was reduced in all four double-blind trials examining the effects of vitamin C, but the reduction was statistically significant in only two of the four, and in some cases reductions were quite modest. Nonetheless, some doctors recommend that people with elevated blood pressure supplement with 1,000 mg vitamin C per day.

Coenzyme Q_{10} (CoQ_{10}) has been reported to affect blood vessels in a way that should cause a decrease in blood pressure.[64] Both uncontrolled and controlled trials have reported that CoQ_{10} significantly lowers blood pressure in people with hypertension.[65,66,67,68,69] All trials used at least 50 mg of CoQ_{10} taken twice per day, and most trials lasted for at least ten weeks.

EPA and DHA, the omega-3 fatty acids found in fish oil, lower blood pressure, according to a metanalysis of 31 trials.[70] That analysis found the effect was dependent on the amount of omega-3 oil used, with the best results occurring in studies using extremely high intakes (15 grams per day). To obtain 15 grams of omega-3s typically requires consumption of 50 grams of fish oil—an unsustainably high amount. Although results with lower intakes were not as impressive, studies using over three grams of omega-3 (generally requiring at least 10 grams of fish oil, or ten 1,000 mg pills per day) also reported significant reduction in blood pressure.

OMEGA-3S & HIGH CHOLESTEROL

Many double-blind studies have consistently demonstrated that fish oils (also called fish-oil concentrates) containing EPA and DHA lower triglyceride levels.[71] The amount of fish oil used in much of the research was an amount that provided 3,000 mg per day of omega-3 fatty acids. To calculate how much omega-3 fatty acid is contained in a fish-oil supplement, add together the amounts of EPA and DHA. For example, a typical 1,000-mg capsule of fish oil provides 180 mg of EPA and 120 mg of DHA (total omega-3 fatty acids = 300 mg). Ten of these capsules would contain

3,000 mg of omega-3 fatty acids. Cod-liver oil, another source of omega-3 fatty acids, has also been found to lower triglycerides.[72]

Omega-3 fatty acids from fish oil and cod-liver oil have been reported to affect blood in many other ways that might lower the risk of heart disease.[73] However, these supplements sometimes increase LDL cholesterol—the bad form of cholesterol. A doctor can check to see if fish oil has this effect on an individual. Research shows that when 900 mg of garlic extract is added to fish oil, the combination still dramatically lowers triglyceride levels but no longer increases LDL cholesterol.[74] Therefore, it appears that taking garlic supplements may be a way to avoid the increase in LDL cholesterol sometimes associated with taking fish oil. People

Fish May Lower Stroke Risk in Men

Recent findings from the Journal of the American Medical Association indicate that men who eat just one serving of fish a month may have a lower risk of the most common type of stroke, which occurs when blood flow to the brain becomes blocked.[77] However, eating more fish may not add much benefit when it comes to lowering the risk of hemorrhagic stroke, which is caused by bleeding in the brain.

A research team led by Dr. Ka He of the Harvard School of Public Health in Boston, Massachusetts observed more than 43,000 men between the ages of 40 and 75 years. They concluded that even though eating fish one to three times a month was associated with a 43 percent lower risk of ischemic stroke, men who reported eating fish at least five times a week were only slightly more protected with a 46 percent lower risk. Exactly how such a small amount of fish, which is rich in omega-3 fatty acids, may lower stroke risk is not clear. However, omega-3 fatty acids may have several different effects on the body, including a reduction in the "stickiness" of platelets, which help form blood clots. Because clots are the cause of 80 percent of strokes, preventing them from forming may ward off strokes.[78] Summarily, Ha and his team suggested "that eating fish once per month or more can reduce the risk of ischemic stroke in men."

Dr. He and his researchers then followed the same men taking part in the Health Professional Follow-up Study, a large national trial. The men in the study, who did not have heart disease or diabetes at the outset, filled out detailed questionnaires about their usual diets. Over the next 12 years, the researchers documented 608 strokes, including 377 ischemic strokes and 106 hemorrhagic strokes. They found no association between omega-3 and the hemorrhagic strokes.

who take fish oil may also need to take vitamin E to prevent the oil from undergoing potentially damaging oxidation in the body.[75] It is not known how much vitamin E is needed to prevent such oxidation; the amount required would presumably depend on the amount of fish oil used. In one study, 300 IU of vitamin E per day prevented oxidation damage in individuals taking 6 grams of fish oil per day.[76]

ANGINA

Chest pain due to reduced blood flow to the heart is known as angina or angina pectoris, and is usually caused by the hardening of the coronary arteries (atherosclerosis) that feed the heart. (Coronary artery spasms may also cause angina.) It is very important that anyone with angina read the section on atherosclerosis; the information there is important for its treatment and prevention. The only items covered here are those that specifically relate to angina.

There are three main types of angina. The first is called stable angina. This type of chest pain comes on during exercise and is both common and predictable. Stable angina is most associated with atherosclerosis. A second type, called variant angina, can occur at rest or during exercise. This type is primarily due to sudden coronary artery spasm, though atherosclerosis may also be a component. The third, most severe type is called unstable angina. It occurs with no predictability and can quickly lead to a heart attack. Anyone with significant, new chest pain or a worsening of previously mild angina must seek medical care immediately.

Fish oils, which contain the beneficial fatty acids known as EPA and DHA, have been studied in the treatment of angina. In some studies, three grams or more of fish oil three times per day (providing a total of about three grams of EPA and two grams of DHA) have reduced chest pain as well as the need for nitroglycerin, a common medication used to treat angina;[79] other investigators could not confirm these findings.[80]

People who take fish oil may also need to take vitamin E to protect the oil from undergoing potentially damaging oxidation in the body.[81] It is not known how much vitamin E is needed to prevent such oxidation; the amount required would presumably depend on the amount of fish oil used. In one study, 300 IU of vitamin E per day prevented oxidation damage in individuals taking six grams of fish oil per day.[82]

SUPPLEMENTS DEMANDED

Omega-3 fatty acids have been part of the human diet for some two to four million years during which our genes were adapting to our environment, including our diets. They are safe and have been listed on the GRAS (Generally Regarded as Safe)

List, according to the FDA. However, today, we are consuming too little of these anti-inflammatory fatty acids and way too much pro-inflammatory omega-6 fatty acids. Our diets must change in order to stave off heart disease, reduce blood pressure, and lower our risk for a heart attack.

Although the AHA says a dietary approach to increasing omega-3 fatty acid intake is preferable, the organization adds in its scientific statement, "for patients with coronary artery disease, the dose of omega-3 (about one gram per day) may be greater than what can readily be achieved through diet alone. These individuals, in consultation with their physician, could consider supplements for CHD risk reduction."

In addition, some types of seafood harbor extremely high levels of mercury and other chlorinated hydrocarbon poisons and consumers should avoid regular consumption. These include shark, swordfish, bluefish and even tuna (which pregnant women, nursing mothers and women planning a pregnancy should limit to no more than once weekly).

Supply your demand for a healthy heart. Take a quality fish oil supplement.

CHAPTER 2

Reduce Cancer Risk
with Omega-3 Fatty Acids

Many Americans have heard of the link between the intake of dietary fats and cardiovascular disease, but few have a good conception of the relationship between the intake of fats and cancer. The relationship is rooted in the fact that what fats we ingest determine the kinds of fats available to the cells; the fatty acids we eat become the building blocks for the three major membranes in the cell membrane and influence the most important properties of the membranes:

- membrane flexibility;
- response of membrane receptors to metabolic compounds (e.g. endocrine hormones);
- kinds of prostaglandins (local tissue hormones) synthesized based on the fatty acids available as raw materials;
- signaling of nuclear DNA by receptors on the cell membrane.

These kinds of influences can have profound effects in the realm of cancer risk and progression.

Omega-3 Fatty Acids and Cancer:
The Laboratory Evidence

For the last two decades evidence that omega-3 fatty acids prevent and intervene in the growth of cancer has been steadily growing; one researcher has written that experiments using either carcinogen-induced or transplanted animal mammary tumor models, as well as in vitro studies, demonstrate that omega-6 polyunsaturated fatty acids (PUFA) promote mammary tumor development more effectively than omega-3 PUFA.[83] (no source in the footnote) Increases in the dietary levels of omega-6 PUFA enhance tumor development, while equivalent increases in dietary levels of omega-3 PUFA often delay or reduce tumor development.

BREAST FRIENDS

Every woman concerned with breast cancer needs to be aware of an amazing landmark study conducted by my professional colleagues, Jeffrey Bland, Ph.D. and Ewan Cameron, M.D., more than a decade ago. Using a special strain of laboratory mouse known for its genetic predisposition for breast cancer, Drs. Bland and Cameron took 350 of these mice and divided them into seven experimental groups of 50 mice each. The control group received only the standard mouse chow as the exclusive dietary source. The remaining six groups were all injected with a known carcinogenic agent. In addition, each of these groups received a different dietary source of fatty acids. One group received ALA and another received EPA. The remaining groups received fatty acids from a variety of vegetable oils commonly consumed by humans in the United States. Neither Bland nor Cameron knew which group received what; only the laboratory technicians knew. Weeks later, the researchers were informed that of the seven groups, two exhibited 100 percent survival and the remaining five groups had 100 percent mortality. Bland and Cameron guessed that one of the survival groups was the control group. They were wrong. To their surprise, all the control animals fed only standard laboratory mouse chow died of the genetically induced breast cancer. The two groups that displayed 100 percent survival, despite genetic cancer risk and injected carcinogens, were the ALA group and EPA groups. All other groups fed typical vegetable oil fatty acids had 100 percent mortality.

These results were so incredible, the editors of the medical journals in which the researchers wanted to publish an article regarding this experiment absolutely insisted that the experiment be repeated. It was, and with the same results. Clearly, this is a strong indication that when we improve the quality of the fatty acids on cell, nuclear, and mitochondrial membranes using omega-3s, we have a powerful beneficial influence on how our cells respond to pathological genetic tendencies and environmental influences.

THE OMEGA-6 PROBLEM

Animal studies suggest that dietary omega-6 fatty acids, found in corn and safflower oils, may be precursors of intermediates involved in the development of mammary tumors. Yet, omega-3s, found in fish oil, can inhibit these effects. A case-control study conducted by UCLA Medical School was designed to examine the relationship between the fatty acid composition of breast adipose (fat) tissue and the risk of breast cancer.[84] Using fatty acid levels in breast tissue as a biomarker of past dietary intake of fatty acids, they examined the hypothesis that breast cancer risk is negatively associated with omega-3 EPA and DHA, and positively associated with omega-6 linoleic acid and arachidonic acid. Breast adipose tissue was collected from 73 breast cancer patients and 74 controls. The linoleic acid and arachidonic acid content was significantly higher in cancer cases than in controls. There was a trend in the data suggesting that, at a given level of omega-6 PUFA, EPA and DHA may have a protective effect. A similar inverse relationship was observed with the omega-3-to-omega-6 ratio. The UCLA team concluded that total omega-6 PUFAs may be contributing to the high risk of breast cancer in the United States and that omega-3 PUFAs, derived from fish oils, may have a protective effect.

THE OMEGA-3 BENEFIT

Experimental studies have indicated that omega-3 fatty acids, including ALA, EPA and DHA, inhibit mammary tumor growth and metastasis. A French laboratory recently examined the fatty acid composition in adipose (fat) tissue from 241 patients with invasive non-metastatic breast carcinoma and from 88 patients with benign breast disease in a case-control study.[85] Again, fatty acid composition in breast adipose tissue was used as a biomarker of past intake of fatty acids. Biopsies were obtained at the time of surgery. Scientists found an inverse association between breast cancer risk and omega-3 fatty acid levels in breast adipose tissue:

- Women with the highest tissue level of ALA had a 61 percent lower risk compared to women at the lowest.
- Women at the highest tissue level of DHA had a 69 percent lower risk than women at the lowest.
- Women at the highest tissue ratio of EPA plus DHA to total omega-6s had a 67 percent lower risk than women at the lowest ratio.

The research team confirmed a protective effect of omega-3 fatty acids on breast cancer risk and supports the hypothesis that the balance between omega-3 and omega-6 fatty acids plays a significant role in breast cancer.

A PALPABLE DIFFERENCE IN THE TISSUES

A Spanish research team focused on tissue omega-3 and omega-6 fatty acid status in the sequence of events from colon polyps to carcinoma.[86] Fatty acid profiles were measured in plasma phospholipids of 22 patients with colorectal cancer, 27 with sporadic polyps, and 12 with normal colon cells (this was the control group). Mucosal fatty acids were measured in the diseased and normal mucosa of cancer and polyps patients, and from the normal mucosa of the control group. There were no differences in fatty acid constituents of plasma phospholipids and normal mucosa between the polyps and control groups, but there were distinctive differences in fatty acids between the diseased and the normal mucosa of the patients in the polyps group. An incremental reduction of EPA concentrations in diseased mucosa from benign adenoma to advanced colon cancer was identified. The diseased mucosa of the cancer patients, in comparison to the normal mucosa, showed lower omega-3s and higher omega-6s. The Spanish team concluded that changes in tissue fatty acid status might participate in the early phases of colorectal cancer in humans.

In another study, researchers at the Catholic University of Rome decided to determine the effect of long-term fish oil supplementation on the rectal mucosal tissue in patients with a history of colon polyps, the precursors of colon cancer. This study involved 60 patients who had just undergone surgery to remove benign colon polyps. The patients were divided into 4 groups. Groups 1, 2, and 3 were supplemented with varying dosages of EPA plus DHA daily, while group 4 received a placebo of olive oil. Biopsy samples from the lower part of the colon lining and blood samples were analyzed at the start of the trial and at the end of the 30-day supplementation period. Patients in the fish oil groups exhibited a significant decrease in tissue arachidonic acid (omega-6) and an increase in tissue EPA and DHA. Concurrently, patients on fish oil experienced a significant decline in the number of abnormal cells in their colon lining compared to the placebo group. Interestingly, reduced tissue proliferation was observed only in patients with abnormal patterns with large numbers of abnormal cells at the beginning of the trial.

The same team conducted a separate six-month study involving 15 polyps patients taking 1.4 grams of EPA and 1.1 grams of DHA daily.[87] The same beneficial effects persisted during long-term, low-dose treatment with no significant side effects. The researchers conclude that low-dose supplementation with fish oils has a normalizing effect on rectal tissue that inhibits the proliferation of abnormal cells, a precursor to polyps. This effect can reduce colon cancer risk.

A WIDE RANGE OF PROTECTIVE EFFECTS

Let's take an overview of the protective effects of omega-3 in the realm of cancer.[88] EPA and DHA have demonstrated protective effects against the following:

- development of carcinogen-induced tumors;
- growth of solid tumors;
- wasting syndrome;
- metastasis in experimental models;
- accelerated proliferation of marker cells in individuals at risk for colon cancer;
- biomarkers of risk for breast cancer.

If a pharmaceutical drug could provide protection against any one of these phenomena without significant side effects, it would be touted as a major breakthrough in cancer care. Omega-3s already can do all of this and more.

HOW CAN OMEGA-3 FATTY ACIDS INFLUENCE CANCER?

Researchers are trying to figure out how omega-3 oils have such a profound desirable effect on cancer cells. For example, results of animal studies have demonstrated that the consumption of omega-3 fatty acids can slow the growth of cancer grafts, increase the efficacy of chemotherapy, and reduce the side effects of chemotherapy or of cancer itself. In prostate cancer cells studied in lab experiments, omega-6 and omega-3 fatty acids have demonstrated promotional and inhibitory effects, respectively. Long-chain omega-3 fatty acids (EPA and DHA) consistently inhibit the growth of human breast cancer cells, both in culture and in grafts applied to immuno-suppressed mice. Dietary intake of omega-3s leads to their incorporation into cell membranes. Increased apoptosis (beneficial cancer cell suicide) in human breast cancer cells following exposure to long-chain omega-3s is generally attributed by scientists to their influence on the tissue enzyme cyclooxygenase-2 (COX-2), which produces various messenger chemicals in nearby tissues called prostaglandins; these influence mammary cancer development. You see, omega-6 fatty acid dominance causes the COX-2 enzyme to produce pro-inflammatory prostaglandins. Omega-3s lead the COX-2 enzyme to produce anti-inflammatory prostaglandins. Meanwhile, we also know that EPA and DHA are likely to activate a chemical with a long complex name—peroxisome proliferator-activated receptor (PPAR)-gamma—which is a key regulator of lipid metabolism and also capable of modulating cancer cell proliferation in a variety of cells including breast cells. Second messenger chemicals including prostaglandins activate the expression of PPAR-gamma in the cell nucleus; under the influence of omega-3s, the PPAR-gamma activation causes apoptosis.[89,90]

Other proposed molecular mechanisms include:

- decreasing the expression of two oncogenes (cancer genes) implicated in tumor promotion;
- inducing differentiation of primordial cancer cells into healthy specialized cells;
- suppressing nuclear factor activation and expression, thus allowing apoptosis of cancer cells;
- reducing cancer-induced cachexia (muscle-wasting).

Based on a substantial body of evidence, researchers conclude that, after appropriate cancer therapy, it is reasonable to consume omega-3 fatty acids in an effort to slow or stop the growth of metastatic cancer cells, increase the longevity of cancer patients, and improve their quality of life.[91]

THE JAPANESE EXPERIENCE

A Japanese study aimed at determining the association between lung cancer and diet involved 748 men and 297 women aged 40 to 79 years who had been diagnosed with lung cancer, and 2,964 male and 1,189 female cancer-free controls.[92] The researchers discovered that men and women who ate cooked or raw fish five or more times weekly had half the incidence of lung cancer, compared to those who ate cooked or raw fish less than once weekly. Women who consumed tofu five or more times weekly had half the risk of cancer, compared to women who consumed tofu less than once weekly. Frequent consumption of carrots was found to be beneficial for women, but detrimental for men, especially smokers. Green vegetables were found to be highly beneficial for men, but not statistically for women. Increased coffee consumption was associated with an increased risk of squamous cell and small cell lung carcinomas in men. Increased consumption of dried or salted fish was not beneficial for men or women. The researchers speculate that processing destroys the beneficial omega-3 oils present in raw and cooked fish.[93]

INCONSISTENT RESULTS

There have been a number of epidemiologic population studies to determine the influence of fish consumption on cancer risk and mortality. Unfortunately, the results have been mixed and contradictory. These results are in stark contrast to the consistently favorable results of laboratory experiments on cell/tissue specimens and animal species. There are some very logical reasons why the population studies have not provided clearly applicable outcomes. Let's take a look at the negative studies.

Japanese people consume significant amounts of long chain omega-3s derived from fish. To study geographic differences in omega-3 intake, a Japanese scientific team compared serum fatty acid and dietary fish intake among various Japanese populations having different rates of cancer mortality. The subjects were 50 men from each of five regions in Japan and 47 Japanese men from Sao Paulo, Brazil. All were randomly selected and aged 40 to 49 years. Serum fatty acids were measured and the frequency of fish intake was obtained via food frequency questionnaires. Significant geographic differences in serum fatty acid levels (percentage of total fatty acids) and fish intake (days per month) were observed. The percentages of serum total polyunsaturated fatty acids were similar in the six regions, though there was an almost three-fold difference in omega-3 content between Brazil (3.9 percent) and Japan (10.9 percent). The frequency of total fish intake corresponded to serum omega-3 composition. The relationship between cancer mortality and serum omega-3 levels was not clear, though an inverse association between prostate cancer and serum omega-3 levels appeared to exist. The results suggest that although serum omega-3s varied significantly, the observed geographic difference did not account for the different cancer risks at the population level.[94]

Another study, based in Sweden, focused on the specific types of fish consumed. Using data from this large, nationwide case-control study, researchers examined the association between consumption of fatty and lean fish and breast cancer risk. High intake of fish was weakly associated with reduced breast cancer risk, but the association was not statistically significant. The calculated risk reduction for women with the highest consumption (3.5 or more servings per week) compared with women with the lowest (virtually none) was only 12 percent. When each type of fish was examined separately, the association was similar for fatty and lean fish.[95]

Intakes of animal protein, meat, and eggs have been associated with breast cancer incidence and mortality in ecological studies, but data from long-term prospective studies are limited. Harvard Medical School and Brigham and Women's Hospital researchers examined these relationships in the Nurses Health Study.[96] They followed 88,647 women for 18 years, with five assessments of diet by food frequency questionnaire, cumulatively averaged and updated over time. During follow-up, 4,107 women developed invasive breast cancer. Compared to the lowest level of intake, the relative risk for the highest level of intake were 1.02 (two percent higher risk) for animal protein, 0.93 (seven percent lower risk) for red meat and 0.89 (11 percent lower risk) for all meat. Results did not differ by menopausal status or family history of breast cancer. The researchers found no evidence that intake of meat or fish during mid-life and later was associated with risk of breast cancer.

Animal studies have, in general, been supportive of the protective effects fish and their omega-3 fatty acids possess against breast cancer risk, but the epidemiologic evidence of such a relationship is limited; case-control and larger studies have rarely shown significant associations. A Danish team investigated among postmenopausal women, in relation to the incidence rate of breast cancer, the association between total fish intake and the effect of fat content and preparation method of the fish.[97] They also investigated the effect of fish intake with respect to estrogen receptor expression of breast cancer tumors. A total of 23,693 postmenopausal women from the prospective study "Diet, Cancer and Health" were included. During follow-up, 424 women were diagnosed with breast cancer. The team's statistical analysis of the data showed, surprisingly, that higher intakes of fish were significantly associated with higher incidence rates of breast cancer. The association was present only for development of estrogen receptor positive breast cancer.

But, before we lose faith in what fish can do for us, let's look at the positive studies.

POSITIVE AND PROVEN

A British research team focused on the ecological association between fat consumption and colorectal and breast cancer risk. Mortality data for breast and colorectal cancer from 24 European nations correlated with the consumption of animal, but not vegetable, fat.[98] There was an inverse correlation with fish and fish oil intake, when expressed as a proportion of total or animal fat. This correlation was significant for colorectal cancer in both genders and for female breast cancer, whether the intakes were current, or 10 years or 23 years before cancer mortality. These effects were only seen in countries with a high animal fat intake. The investigators concluded that fish oil consumption is associated with protection against the promotional effects of animal fat in colorectal and breast cancer. In their opinion, a 15 percent decrease in animal fat intake combined with a three-fold increase in fish oil intake could reduce male colon cancer risk by 30 percent in countries with a high animal fat intake. The desired three-fold increase in fish oil intake could be achieved by eating fish three times a week or by taking two standard fish oil capsules daily.

Data from a series of case-control studies, conducted in Italy and Switzerland between 1991 and 2001, have been analyzed by Italian scientists to evaluate the role of omega-3 fatty acid intake in the development of cancers in the oral cavity and pharynx (736 cases, 1,772 controls); esophagus (395 cases, 1,066 controls); large bowel (1,394 colon, 886 rectum, 4,765 controls); breast (2,900 cases, 3,122 controls); and ovary (1,031 cases, 2,411 controls).[99] The controls were patients admitted to hospital for acute, non-cancerous conditions, unrelated to modifications in diet. The cancer risk for the highest intake of omega-3s, compared to the lowest, were 50 percent less for oral and pharyngeal cancer; 50 percent less for esophageal cancer; 30 percent less for colon cancer; 20 percent less for rectal and breast cancer; and 40 percent less for ovarian cancer. The risk benefits were significant for all cancer sites, excluding rectal and breast cancer. These results suggest that omega-3 PUFAs decrease the risk of several cancers.

COLORECTAL CANCER

United Kingdom public health officials studied the relationship between omega-3s and certain forms of cancer.[100] Mortality data for breast and colorectal cancer in 24 European countries were correlated with current fish and fish oil consumption and with consumption 10 and 23 years previously. In males, there was an inverse correlation between colorectal cancer mortality and current intake of fish, a weaker correlation with fish consumption 10 years earlier and none with consumption 23 years earlier. Investigators concluded that fish consumption is associated with protection against the later promotional stages of colorectal cancer progression, but not with the early initiation stages.

Japanese researchers conducted a large case-reference study with 928 cases of colon cancer, 622 of rectal cancer, and 46,886 cancer-free outpatient controls aged 40 to 79 years.[101] The data showed frequent raw/cooked fish intake to be associated with decreased risk for male colon cancer, especially for males over age 60, smokers, and frequent meat-eaters. A marginal decrease in risk was also detected for female rectal cancer, especially in the regular physical exercise subgroup. Frequent dried/salted fish intake increased risk in females younger than 60 and alcohol drinkers. The results suggest that frequent raw/cooked fish intake may decrease the risk, while dried/salted fish may exert a detrimental effect.

BREAST CANCER

Finally, we have convincing human evidence that levels of various fatty acids in adipose breast tissue and the emergence of aggressive metastases are intimately related.[102] The Yale University School of Medicine conducted a recent case-control study to investigate the association between intake of fatty acids and breast cancer risk.[103] Data from 1,119 women (565 cases and 554 controls) were used. Dietary information was obtained through a food-frequency questionnaire. In the full study population, there were no significant trends for any fatty acid when comparing the highest to the lowest levels of intake. Among pre-menopausal women, consumption of the highest compared with the lowest quartile of the omega-3/omega-6 ratio was associated with a significantly lower risk of breast cancer. The Yale team concluded that a higher ratio might reduce the risk of breast cancer, especially in premenopausal women.

PROSTATE CANCER

Can high consumption of fish and marine fatty acids reduce the risk of prostate cancer? Strongly so, according to the Department of Nutrition, Harvard School of Public Health, which followed 47,882 men participating in the Health Professionals Follow-up Study.[105] Dietary intake was assessed in 1986, 1990, and 1994 using a validated food frequency questionnaire. During 12 years of follow-ups, 2,482 cases of prostate cancer were diagnosed, of which 617 were advanced, including 278 metastatic cases. Eating fish more than three times per week was associated with a reduced risk of prostate cancer and the strongest association was for metastatic cancer. Intake of marine fatty acids from food showed a similar but weaker association. Each additional daily intake of 0.5 gm of marine fatty acid from food was associated with a 24 percent decrease in risk of metastatic prostate cancer. Men with high consumption of fish had a lower risk of prostate cancer, especially for metastatic types (those that spread from one organ throughout the body). Marine fatty acids may account for part of the effect, but other factors in fish may also play a role.

In the meantime, men concerned about prostate health are advised to reduce their intake of red meat, while increasing intake of a broad range of fresh, organic

FYI: Life-saving Information
Omega-3s Inhibit Breast Cancer Metastasis

In a study published in the *British Journal of Cancer,* 121 women patients with an initially localized breast cancer were studied.[104] Their breast adipose tissue was obtained at the time of initial surgery and its fatty acid content analyzed. A low level of alpha-linolenic acid (found predominantly in flax) was strongly associated with the presence of vascular invasion, indicating the cancer was likely to spread. After an average 31 months of follow-up, 21 patients developed metastases. Large tumor size, high cell-division rates, presence of vascular invasion and low levels of alpha-linolenic acid were single factors significantly associated with an increased risk of metastasis. The take-home message from this study is clear: optimal levels of flax and its omega-3 fatty acids can reduce risk of breast cancer spread.

These studies support the work of French researchers who recently found that low levels of the omega-3 fatty acid alpha-linolenic acid could predict the increased risk of breast cancer. The study was published in the February 2000 issue of the *European Journal of Cancer.* This case-control study conducted in central France was designed to explore whether alpha-linolenic acid inhibits breast cancer, using fatty acid levels in breast adipose (fat) tissue as an indication of its intake. Biopsies of breast adipose tissue at the time of diagnosis were obtained from 123 women with invasive non-metastatic breast carcinoma, while 59 women with benign breast disease served as controls. Women with the highest levels of alpha-linolenic acid experienced a 74 percent reduced risk for breast cancer, compared with those women with the lowest intake. According to the researchers, the results suggest "a protective effect of alpha-linolenic acid in the risk of breast cancer."

foods. Be sure to take a high-potency vitamin-mineral supplement with zinc daily and use fish oils.[106,107,108,109,110,111]

LUNG CANCER

Omega-3 fatty acids in fish oil exhibit a variety of health benefits, and there is evidence that they can inhibit the development of human lung carcinomas. To examine the hypothesis that fish consumption reduces the risk of lung cancer, a Japanese team conducted a population-based prospective study, following 5,885 residents for 14 years.[112] A total of 51 incident lung cancer cases were observed, and they found a clear decreasing relative risk for lung cancer with increased frequency of consumption of fish and shellfish, but not with intake of dried/salted fish. Decreased relative risk was seen with broiling and boiling cooking methods, but reduction with raw and deep-fried fish consumption was not statistically significant. The scientists concluded that frequent fresh fish consumption, regardless of cooking method, may reduce the risk of lung cancer.

PANCREATIC CANCER

Because a number of polyunsaturated fatty acids have been shown to inhibit the growth of malignant cells in lab experiments, researchers investigated whether fatty acids modify the growth of human pancreatic cancer. To do so, they studied lauric, stearic, palmitic, oleic, linoleic, alpha-linolenic, gamma-linolenic, arachidonic, docosahexaenoic (DHA) and eicosapentaenoic (EPA) acids and the effect of each fatty acid on cell growth.[113] All the polyunsaturated fatty acids tested had an inhibitory effect, with EPA (found in fish and formed from alpha-linolenic acid in flax) being the most potent. Monounsaturated (e.g., olive oil) or saturated fatty acids (found in beef and dairy) were not inhibitory.

According to the report, "The ability of certain fatty acids to inhibit significantly the growth of three human pancreatic cancer cell lines in vitro (within an artifical environment) at concentrations which could be achieved in vivo (within the body) suggests that administration of such fatty acids may be of therapeutic benefit in patients with pancreatic cancer." In this case, fish, with its rich source of preformed EPA, may prove to be cancer preventive with flax exhibiting significant, yet lesser, inhibitory properties.

HIDDEN GREMLINS THAT CONFOUND THE RESULTS

Some researchers have been puzzled by some inconsistencies in lab experiments exploring the effect of omega-3s on cancer. Questions have also arisen about inconsistencies in epidemiological studies. In population studies, high fish intake over many years is associated with reduced risks of breast and colorectal cancer. Prospective and case-control studies either do not show an association between fish intake and cancer risk or show reduced risk at high fish intakes. What may be the reasons for these discrepancies?

With respect to lab experiments, some scientists have addressed this issue by looking at hidden factors that must be taken into account. The effects omega-3 fatty acids have on tumor growth depend upon the background levels of omega-6 fatty acids and antioxidants. Variations in these compounds may account for previously inconsistent results in experimental carcinogenesis.[114] This factor not only applies to lab experiments; it also applies to epidemiological studies of population groups.

A number of factors may have been overlooked by designers of epidemiological studies:

- There has generally been no accounting for background omega-6 intake that would affect fatty acid ratios.
- There has been no accounting for antioxidant status.
- There has been little accounting for concurrent meat intake, a major source of omega-6 if the animals are grain-fed. The positive link between certain cancers and meat intake may suggest the influence of animal hormones and fatty acids produced from grain consumption by livestock.
- No distinction is made between wild fish, richer in natural omega-3s, and farm fish, raised on man-made fish food rich in omega-6s.
- No distinction is made between freshwater and saltwater fish, between fish from cold Arctic waters or those from warmer regions. These factors influence omega-3 content.
- In addition to adding omega-3s to our daily routine, cancer risk might be reduced even more effectively when wild fish is used to replaced high-saturated fat meals.

There has even been a clinical study design artifact overlooked by some researchers. Some of the study literature on the clinical efficacy of fish oil has been equivocal. This may be due to the erroneous selection of olive oil as a placebo. The concept of double blind, placebo-controlled crossover research requires the selection of placebo substances known to be biologically inert. Olive oil is not biologically inert; in fact, it is known to have its own health-benefiting effects, especially in the realm of cardiovascular health where fish oil is also operative. Therefore, the use of olive oil as a placebo relative to fish oil may mask the beneficial effects of fish oil.[115]

Taking all these factors into consideration, the preponderance of evidence indicates that incorporation of wild fish and fresh, pure omega-3 oils into our eating habits provides significant protection against cancer.

HELP FOR CACHEXIA
(ABNORMAL WEIGHT LOSS FROM MUSCLE WASTING)

Severe weight loss with muscle wasting is one of the debilitating aspects of cancer. Safe, non-toxic ways of preventing or slowing this disabling process can be of great value to cancer patients. Although omega-3 fatty acids are not magic bullets in this regard, they should be considered as part of an overall nutritional regimen for patients enduring this malignancy.

Based on results of previous studies suggesting that administering EPA will stabilize weight in patients with advanced pancreatic cancer, researchers at the Royal Infirmary of Edinburgh decided to determine if a combination of EPA with a conventional oral nutritional supplement could produce weight gain in these patients. 20 patients with inoperable pancreatic adenocarcinoma were asked to consume two cans of a fish oil-enriched nutritional supplement daily, in addition to normal food intake. Each can contained 310 calories, 16.1 grams of protein and 1.09 grams of EPA. Patients were assessed for weight, body composition, dietary intake, resting energy expenditure (REE) and performance status. They also consumed a median of 1.9 cans daily. All patients were losing weight at the start of the trial at an average rate of 2.9 kg (about 6.4 lbs) monthly. After administration of the fish oil-enriched supplement, patients had significant weight-gain at both three (average 1 kg, or 2.2 lbs) and seven weeks (average 2 kg, or 4.4 lbs). Dietary intake increased significantly by almost 400 calories per day. Performance status and appetite were significantly improved after three weeks. In contrast to previous studies, this study suggests that an EPA-enriched supplement may not only slow or stop wasting away in general; it may even reverse wasting in advanced pancreatic and, perhaps other cancers. The researchers concluded that a fish oil-enriched nutritional supplement may be a safe and effective means of preventing weight loss in cancer patients and may even increase survival time in patients with pancreatic cancer.[116]

For patients with end-stage cancer, chemotherapy and other conventional interventions have been problematic for their quality of life, and less than impressive in terms of treatment. A Greek research team conducted a prospective, randomized control study to investigate the effect of dietary omega-3 fatty acids plus vitamin E on the immune status and survival of well-nourished and malnourished patients with generalized malignancy.[117] Sixty patients with generalized solid tumors were randomized to receive dietary supplements with either fish oil (18 grams of omega-3 fatty acids) or a placebo daily until death. Each group included 15 well-nourished and 15 malnourished patients. The scientists measured total T-cells, T-helper cells, T-suppressor cells, natural killer cells, and the synthesis of chemical messengers by peripheral white blood cells before and on the 40th day of fish oil supplementation. The research team followed all patients until they died. The ratio of T-helper cells to T-suppressor cells was significantly lower in malnourished patients. Omega-3 fatty acids increased this ratio in the subgroup of malnourished patients. There were no significant differences in chemical messenger production among the various groups, except for a decrease in tumor necrosis factor production in malnourished cancer patients, which was restored by omega-3 fatty acids. The average survival time was significantly higher for the subgroup of well-nourished patients in both groups. Malnourished patients had a much shorter survival time than the well nourished (an average of 213 days versus 481 days). But omega-3 fatty acids prolonged survival among all patients. Both malnourished and well-nourished patients who received fish oil and vitamin E survived significantly longer than did patients on placebo. The Greek researchers concluded that malnutrition could be a predictor of survival for patients with end-stage malignancy. Omega-3 fatty acids, especially those in fish oil, seem to have a modulating effect on the immune system and to prolong the survival of malnourished patients with generalized malignancy.

CHAPTER 3

Omega-3s for Mental Health

There isn't a person living today who won't benefit from omega-3 fatty acids. However, persons suffering from depression, alcoholism, attention deficit disorder, impulsive and violent behavior, or emotional hostility can particularly benefit by favoring omega-3 fatty acids in their diet. In some of the most amazing research done today, scientists have discovered that the type of fat one consumes is "inextricably linked with your state of mind."[118]

Beyond Prozac and St. John's wort, omega-3 fatty acids may be an excellent supplement for persons suffering from depression, hostility or violent, self-destructive behavior. No matter whether the depressed person utilizes fluoxetine (Prozac), St. John's wort or other synthetic or natural medicines, one will never truly overcome many mood disorders without adequate intake of omega-3 fatty acids. It may be extraordinary to think but is truthful to say these essential fats appear to be as important as medical drugs or natural medicines when it comes to relieving mood disorders.

The brain is comprised of 77 percent water and 10 to12 percent lipids (fats). However, this isn't the kind of fat found in the area of the abdomen, thighs or buttocks. This is structural fat that forms cell membranes and governs cellular function. What's more, the nerve cells of the brain, in a state of optimal nutrition, are extremely rich in omega-3 fatty acids. In fact, the brain's nerve cells contain five times more omega-3 fatty acids than red blood cells. However, the modern Western diet is severely depleted in omega-3 fatty acids. Thus, the nerve cells of persons with mood disorders may be starved of this essential fat.

LIFESTYLE CHANGES FOR THE WORSE

Depression seems to have increased continuously since the beginning of the century. It is now one of the most commonly diagnosed conditions in the world. A contributing factor is the change in Western eating habits, in which omega 3 fatty acids contained in wild fish, wild game and vegetables has been replaced by omega-6 fatty acids of cereal grain oils.

A LOOK AT THE EVIDENCE ON FATTY ACIDS AND MOOD

A recent review of the literature indicates that all studies on major depression revealed either a significant decrease of the polyunsaturated omega-3 fatty acids, an increase of the omega-6/omega-3 ratios in plasma, in the membranes of the red cells. In addition, two studies found a higher severity of depression when the level of polyunsaturated omega-3 fatty acids or the omega-3/omega-6 ratio was low.

Low-fat diets have been widely promoted for lowering cholesterol levels, for reducing body weight, and for preventing certain types of cancer. At least one study, however, has found that although a reduction in cholesterol may reduce mortality from heart disease, it may increase the incidence of fatal accidents, violent deaths, suicides, and depression.

Researchers at the University of Arizona now believe that they may have found an explanation for this phenomenon.[121] They point out that fat restriction and cholesterol-lowering drugs may change the concentrations of polyunsaturated fatty acids in the tissues including nerve tissue (neurons). Fat-restricting diets usually lead to a relative increase in the intake of omega-6s and a relative decrease in the intake of omega-3 fatty acids. This can have serious consequences inasmuch as the omega-3 fatty acids EPA and DHA are crucial for the proper functioning of the nervous system.

Epidemiologic studies have found a clear correlation between a low intake of EPA and DHA and the prevalence of depression; these indicate a clear association between low blood levels of EPA and DHA and an increased risk of depression, violence and suicide. A recent study in Japan found that DHA supplementation reduced aggression among healthy Japanese students. Two other Japanese studies found that

Did You Know?
The Omega-3-5-HIAA Connection

Here's why omega-3 fatty acids profoundly affect mood. Serotonin is a brain neurotransmitter that plays a key role in keeping people happy. Optimal levels of serotonin are essential to feeling good. Severely depressed patients, however, are known to have very low levels of a serotonin metabolite or breakdown product known as 5-HIAA (5-hydroxyindoleacetic acid). It is now known that essential fatty acid levels in the body predict 5-HIAA levels (and probably in turn, serotonin levels). [119,120]

the incidence of depression was only 0.9 percent and 0 percent and the intake of EPA plus DHA was 1.5 grams per day and 4.2 grams per day, respectively. On the other hand, two studies of population groups in the United States found that the incidence of depression was 3.7 percent and 2.9 percent. The average intake of EPA and DHA in the U.S. is estimated to be about 0.1 gram per day.

Other studies have shown that on-off dieting can produce a serious imbalance in the ratio of fatty acids and may lead to depression. The researchers conclude that an extremely low-fat diet may be counter-productive and have deleterious psychological ramifications. They stress that dietary advice regarding cholesterol reduction, weight loss, and cancer prevention should emphasize the importance of an adequate intake of omega-3 fatty acids.

HOW DO OMEGA-3S AFFECT MOOD?

DHA found in fish oil is the building block of human brain tissue membranes. It is particularly abundant in the gray matter of the brain and the retina. Brain membranes naturally have a very high content in essential fatty acids for which they depend on dietary sources. Any dietary lack of essential fatty acids adversely affects cerebral development, modifies the activity of enzymes of cerebral membranes, and decreases learning ability.

The omega-3 fatty acids are incorporated into the membrane phospholipids of nerve cells (neurons). DHA is essential to neurological functions. According to one research team, "Docosahexaenoic acid (DHA) with 22-carbons and 6 double bonds is the extreme example of an omega-3 polyunsaturated fatty acid (PUFA)." One of DHA's unique features is its conformational flexibility that multiple double bonds are known to confer. DHA significantly alters many basic properties of membranes including "fluidity," behavior, elastic compressibility, permeability, fusion, and protein activity. "DHA's interaction with other membrane lipids, particularly cholesterol, may play a prominent role in modulating the local structure and function of cell membranes."[122]

Interaction between neurons arises from the rapid synthesis, release and degradation of chemical messengers (neurotransmitters). Response to neurotransmitter communication depends on neuron membrane integrity and responsiveness. The fact that DHA is a principal component of nerve cell membranes means that DHA deficits will lead to nervous system dysfunction. In addition, as with all nutritional matters, the biochemical individuality of the patient is paramount. The unique needs of the individual patient must be met in order to achieve gratifying results.

The value of DHA for the development of the central nervous system during fetal development and during infancy is well established. Since the nervous tissue of the retina of the eye is an extension of the nervous system, optimal retinal development during pregnancy and infancy also require optimal DHA nutrition. Ideally, the DHA content of an infant's brain triples during the first three months of life. Low levels of DHA have been linked to depression, memory loss, dementia, and visual problems in later years.

An additional beneficial effect of omega-3s involves inflammation. In major depression, the inflammatory response system is activated, resulting in elevated pro-inflammatory cytokines (white blood cell chemical messengers) and eicosanoids (fatty acid derivatives, such as prostaglandin E_2) in the blood and the cerebrospinal fluid of depressed patients. These substances trigger peroxidation, damaging membrane phospholipids, including those containing polyunsaturated fatty acids. The cytokines and eicosanoids are manufactured from polyunsaturated fatty acids and have opposite functions according to their precursors are omega- 3 or omega-6. Arachidonic acid (omega-6) is converted into pro-inflammatory prostaglandin E_2 (PGE_2); omega-3 fatty acids inhibit the formation of PGE_2. Dietary increase in omega-3 fatty acids reduces strongly the production of pro-inflammatory compounds.[123]

ESSENTIAL FATTY ACIDS FOR ALMOST EVERY COMMON MOOD DISORDER

Could it be that essential fatty acid levels play a role in almost all of our most common mood disorders? The preliminary evidence is convincing. Let's take a closer look.

Depression

In depression, there is strong epidemiological evidence that fish consumption reduces the risk of becoming depressed and evidence that cell membrane levels of omega-3s are reduced.

Our first clue comes from research that has found the lowest rates of depression worldwide seem to be correlated with the amount of fish consumed per capita.[124] Decreased omega-3 fatty acid consumption correlates with increasing rates of depression. Geographic areas where consumption of DHA is high are associated with decreased rates of depression. DHA deficiency states (alcoholism and the post-partum period) are linked to depression. Persons with major depression are tissue-depleted in omega-3 fatty acids, especially DHA.[125] Of course, fish is one of the prime sources of omega-3 fatty acids. It is also known that depressed patients have very low levels of the omega-3 fatty acid EPA in their serum and red blood cells.

Cutting edge research has also recently pinpointed among depressed persons marked depletions of omega-3 fatty acids in the phospholipid membranes of red blood cells (which are thought to hold similar fatty acid concentrations as in nerve cell membranes).[126,127,128] Adipose (fat tissue) DHA is a measure of long-term dietary intake. Human studies indicate that the higher the adipose tissue DHA levels, the lower the incidence of depression.[129]

Postpartum Depression

The tragic recent news reports that postpartum depression drove a Texas mother to slay her five children brings this often-overlooked condition into the spotlight. This mood disorder may be linked to omega-3 and other nutritional deficiencies. Bearing and nursing children puts enormous nutritional demands on mothers' bodies. They must eat a diet that is sufficiently abundant in macronutrients (protein, fats, and complex carbohydrates) and micronutrients (vitamins, minerals, and other nutritional factors) to adequately meet the needs of her hard-working body, as well as that of her child. Because breast-feeding women are passing on their essential fatty acids to their newborns, it is quite common for nursing mothers to deplete their own omega-3 fatty acid stores; therefore, it is critical that women who are pregnant or lactating receive adequate omega-3s in food or supplements. Though fish is a great source, many women avoid seafood during pregnancy due to high toxic chemical contamination in many such species.

Omega-3 fatty acids are essential to the normal brain development of the newborn, especially during the last three months of pregnancy, when the brain of the unborn baby increases in size threefold, notes Dr. Simopolous. If women neglect to take in enough essential fatty acids, the priorities of nature will cause the unborn baby to receive these nutrients from the mother's tissues. Even the mother's limited supplies still may not be enough to meet baby's needs optimally; modern laboratory testing shows new mothers have only half the normal blood levels of omega-3 fatty acids.[130] The lesson is clear: all pregnant and nursing women should consider supplementation with purified fish oils or flax.

No wonder it used to be common practice for women to take cod liver oil during pregnancy! Scientists at the Mayo Clinic note, "The mental apparatus of the coming generation is developed in [the womb] and the time to begin supplementation is before conception. A normal brain cannot be made without an adequate supply of omega-3 fatty acids, and there may be no later opportunity to repair the effects of an omega-3 fatty acid deficiency once the nervous system is formed."[131]

Impulsive, Violent Behavior

There are many theories on the link between diet and the environment and anti-social behavior. Genetics and environmental poisoning with lead, manganese, and other contaminants are two influences linked to violent behavior. However, studies indicate that essential fatty acids play an important role. One study found that violent criminals have much lower levels of a type of omega-3 fatty acids than persons without a history of violence.[132] "A similar phenomenon has been observed in primates," notes Dr. Simopolous. "Feeding male money monkeys a diet with a high ratio of omega-6 to omega-3 fatty acids (33:1) has resulted in more slapping, grappling, pushing, and biting."[133]

Another study showed that normal people given omega-3 fatty acids can also reduce their hostility level as a result of the stresses of daily life, adds Dr. Simopolous. In this study, Japanese scientists gave either omega-3 fatty acids or a placebo to college students. During examination week, students given the natural medicine exhibited much more measured goodwill, compared to those receiving the placebo who scored higher on tests designed to measure hostility.[134]

Persons with a history of violent, impulsive behaviors and those with non-violent behavior were studied for their levels of DHA. Violent persons had significantly higher lifetime violence and hostility ratings and lower concentrations of 5-HIAA than nonviolent subjects, according to research from the Laboratory of Membrane Biochemistry and Biophysics, National Institute on Alcohol Abuse and Alcoholism in Bethesda, Maryland. There may be a correlation between plasma DHA levels and violent behavior.[135]

A recent Japanese double-blind, placebo-controlled study was conducted to see if DHA can reduce aggression against others among people aged 50-60 years. It is interesting that among villagers living a more rural, agrarian lifestyle, there was no significant difference between the control and DHA groups in aggression. Yet, DHA favorably controlled aggression among white-collar workers. Perhaps DHA is of particular benefit among those living the modern high-tech, high-stress lifestyle. The daily intake of 150 to 160 mg daily of DHA was not enough to control aggression. A dosage of 1.5gm DHA daily is needed to achieve desired results.[136]

Oxford University scientists examined evidence that criminal offenders consume diets lacking in essential nutrients and surmised that this state of sub-optimal nutrition could adversely affect their behavior. To test empirically whether adequate intakes of vitamins, minerals and essential fatty acids could reduce anti-social behavior, the Oxford team designed a double-blind, placebo-controlled, randomized trial of nutritional supplements involving 231 young adult prison inmates. The Oxford investigators compared the rate and type of disciplinary offences before and during supplementation. Those receiving active nutrients committed an average of 26.3 percent fewer offences, whereas placebos remained essentially unchanged. The Oxford team concluded that anti-social behavior in prisons, including violence, could be reduced by vitamins, minerals and essential fatty acids.[137]

The implications for those eating poor diets in the community are similar. Moreover, for a society spending a fortune daily to house more than a million prisoners, the ramifications and possibilities arising from this research on violent behavior are staggering. One wonders how much money and human misery could be saved through an enlightened application of understanding how good nutrition can rehabilitate people's lives.

Bipolar Disorders

Researchers at Brigham and Women's Hospital and the Department of Psychiatry of Harvard Medical School believe that omega-3 fatty acids may inhibit neuronal signal pathways in a manner similar to that of lithium carbonate and valproate, which are two effective pharmaceuticals for bipolar disorder. A four-month, double-blind study using 30 bipolar patients was conducted to examine whether omega-3 fatty acids exhibit mood-stabilizing properties in bipolar disorder. The omega-3 fatty acid group, which took 9.6 gm of omega-3 daily, had a significantly longer period of remission than the controls using a placebo of olive oil. And most gratifyingly, "for nearly every other outcome measure, the omega-3 fatty acid group performed better than the placebo group." The Harvard team concluded that omega-3 fatty acids were well tolerated and improved the short-term course of illness.[138]

A very recent study sought to determine if greater seafood consumption, considered by the authors as a measure of omega-3 fatty acid intake, is linked to lower rates of bipolar disorder in samples of community populations. Lifetime prevalence rates in various countries for bipolar disorders and schizophrenia were identified from population-based epidemiological studies. Statistical analyses compared prevalence data to differences in apparent seafood consumption. The investigators found that greater seafood consumption predicted lower lifetime prevalence rates of bipolar disorders. It is interesting that bipolar II disorder and bipolar spectrum disorder have a vulnerability threshold below 50 pounds of seafood per person per year. There was no noted correlation between lifetime prevalence rates of schizophrenia and seafood consumption. The researchers felt they had discovered a "robust correlation relationship between greater seafood consumption and lower prevalence rates of bipolar disorders. These data provide a cross-national context for understanding ongoing clinical intervention trials of omega-3 fatty acids in bipolar disorders."[139]

Schizophrenia

After treating some 26 patients with chronic mental illness for ten years or more, Dr. Abram Hoffer in 1993 reported on his results.[140] While under conventional therapy, around five percent of schizophrenic patients may experience significant gains in mental health. However, in his small clinical study, by utilizing omega-3 oils in addition to other nutritional supplements, some eighteen patients could go on to function normally in the everyday world: three improved greatly; five moderately; and one, not at all.

A British team recently looked at the connection between fatty acids and schizophrenia. Evidence supporting the role of fatty acids in schizophrenia includes abnormal brain phospholipid turnover, increased levels of phospholipase A(2) (the enzyme which extricates fatty acids from cell membranes for conversion into local hormones called protaglandins), reduced niacin skin flush response, and reduced cell membrane levels of omega-3 and omega-6 fatty acids. Four out of five placebo-controlled double-blind trials of EPA in the treatment of schizophrenia have given positive findings. What role EPA plays is currently not known, but arachidonic acid (omega-6) is important in schizophrenia. These investigators are convinced that clinical improvement using EPA treatment correlates with membrane changes in arachidonic acid.

A research group in India supplemented 33 patients for four months with a mixture of EPA/DHA (180:120 mg) and antioxidants (vitamin E/C, 400 IU:500 mg) each morning and evening. The red blood cell (RBC) membrane fatty acid levels, plasma lipid peroxides and clinical measures were carried at pre-treatment, post-treatment, and after four months of post-supplementation period to determine the stability of therapeutic effects. Levels of fatty acids and lipid peroxides were compared with their levels in normal controls. As expected, post-treatment levels of RBC fatty acids were significantly higher than pre-treatment levels, while levels in the normal controls had no significant increase. Furthermore, there was a significant reduction in mental dysfunction based on psychiatric tests and an increase in the quality of life measures. The fatty acid levels returned to pretreatment levels after four months of washout. Nevertheless, clinical improvement was remarkably retained.

Alzheimer's Disease

The mental deterioration of Alzheimer's disease is not only devastating to patients, it is also catastrophic for the entire family. Although omega-3 fatty acids do not constitute a cure for this dreaded condition, they can offer some assistance in slowing the disease and improving the patients' quality of life.

Several scientific papers have indicated the value of omega-3 oils for Alzheimer's patients.[141]

Scottish researchers found plasma and blood cell levels of essential fatty acids to be abnormal among patients with this disorder. They conducted a small double-blind, placebo-controlled trial with 36 patients taking fatty acids and antioxidants for 20 weeks. The investigators found the fatty acid/antioxidant combination to be superior to the placebo in improving the status of these patients.

American research has found that in Alzheimer's disease, the production of pro-inflammatory compounds, which are damaging to cerebral blood vessels, is a major component of the onset of the malady. This irreversible brain disorder may be caused by fundamentally important inflammatory processes associated with aging, and not, as generally believed, by plaque-like deposits in the brain (which might be secondary to the inflammation), report scientists in the April 2001 issue of *Trends in Neurosciences*.[142] In this regard, we note the low incidence of Alzheimer's among the elderly in Japan. Because the fatty acids in fish oil are known to inhibit the synthesis of these inflammatory compounds, researchers have proposed the use of fish oil as part of a regimen to slow the progression of Alzheimer's during early stages.[143]

THE DOCTORS' PRESCRIPTION FOR
IMPROVED MOODS & WELL BEING

If you have any problems maintaining a positive mood, get a professional diagnosis from an open-minded provider. If necessary, educate that person about the value of omega-3 fatty acids in mental health. Then incorporate them into your diet in moderate doses. Clearly, the conventional medical community needs to become more aware of the link between omega-3 fatty acids and mood—and the extreme value of omega-3 fatty acids in mental health.

For most of us who seek to simply improve our mood and mental outlooks, we can safely increase our intake of omega-3 fatty acids. Consider taking fish oil capsules daily or consuming wild fish particularly rich in these essential fatty acids, two to three times weekly. Such sources include wild Pacific salmon, rainbow trout, tuna, sardines, and mackerel.

CHAPTER 4

Omega-3s–Rescuing ADHD Children & Adults

Lines form on my face and hands/Lines form from the ups and downs
I'm in the middle without any plans/I'm a boy and I'm a man
I'm eighteen and I don't know what I want
Eighteen I just don't know what I want/Eighteen I gotta get away
I gotta get out of this place/I'll go runnin' in outer space
Oh yeah/I got a baby's brain and an old man's heart
Took eighteen years to get this far
Don't always know what I'm talkin' about
Feels like I'm livin' in the middle of doubt/Cause I'm Eighteen
I get confused every day/Eighteen/I just don't know what to say
Eighteen/I gotta get away
—Alice Cooper, "I'm Eighteen"

Impulsiveness. Inattentiveness. Hyperactivity. We all know the warning signs that often are the prelude to school officials diagnosing children with attention deficit/hyperactivity disorder (ADHD).

Is your child on Ritalin? Do school officials want you to put your child on Ritalin because of his or her poor behavior, lack of concentration, or lack of learning skills?

Although teachers and school officials often are ones who attempt to diagnose children with ADHD, parents should always make the final decision, in consultation with a professional specializing in this field, as to whether the child will be medicated. It is essential that parents make a decision that is in the child's best short- and long-term interest. For some children, drug therapies may be appropriate. But, for others, drug therapy may lead to potential complications, including increased risk for adult behavioral disorders, drug abuse, criminal activity, and possibly even growth inhibition and cancer (since Ritalin has shown some evidence of carcinogenicity). Drug therapy is the course of last resort when all else has failed. In the meantime, many contributing factors must be first identified and eliminated beforehand. These include food additives, refined carbohydrates, and food allergies.

Attention deficit/hyperactivity disorder can be tragic for children so diagnosed, as well as their families. Conventional wisdom is of the view that, in most children with ADHD, the cause is biological and multifactorial. Yet on deeper reflection, this disorder seems even bizarre. Human beings have been raising their offspring on Earth for thousands of years. During all this time it was not necessary to drug children into appropriate behavior. Why now? And why is it happening only in Western industrialized societies, particularly the United States?

It is intriguing that some researchers have found that children with ADHD were breast-fed less often as infants than were children free of ADHD. Breast milk contains DHA in amounts varying with the mother's intake of omega-3 fatty acids. Unfortunately, the average DHA content of breast milk in the United States is the lowest in the world, probably because Americans eat relatively little small amounts of wild fish, wild game, or livestock raised on green vegetation. Amazingly, the United States is the only country in the world where infant formulas are not required to be fortified with DHA, despite World Health Organization recommendations to do so. Is it possible that ADHD and poor academic performance in the United States are linked to DHA deficiency? If this is true, then we are producing generations of young Americans ill-equipped to meet the challenges of the future due to an easily correctable nutritional deficit.

MEDICATING GENERATION RX

We used to call the post-boomer generation Generation X. Now we are raising Generation Rx. As a recent national magazine says, "Drugs have become increasingly popular for treating kids with mood and behavior problems. But how will that affect them in the long run?"

One of the authors (Dr. Joiner-Bey) is acquainted with someone who supervised children of middle (junior high) school age attending a summer educational enrichment program at a private college in New England. The vast majority of these kids came from very affluent parents who could afford to give their children the advantage of this kind of exclusive opportunity. Amazingly, one-third of the group of otherwise healthy youngsters arrived at the college with strict medication instructions for daily doses of Ritalin (methylphenidate). To our acquaintance, the sight of children from socio-economically advantaged backgrounds, lining up to receive their daily dose of mind-altering drug, was as weird as something out of science fiction. It

Did You Know?
Baby Formulas Deficient
in Omega-3 Fatty Acids

It is now well understood that DHA, the 22-carbon omega-3 fatty acid, is essential to the healthy development of nervous tissue in infants and children. In healthy, well-nourished adults, the major repository of DHA in the body is the nervous system, including the brain and the neurons of the retina of eye. The importance of omega-3 fatty acids in nervous system growth, development, and functioning has become a central issue in the production of infant formulas. The majority of infant formulas are nearly devoid of omega-3 fatty acids, while loaded with omega-6 fatty acids. Infants who receive adequate omega-3 fatty acids score higher on aptitude tests and have better visual acuity. This is one of the reasons that mother's milk is thought to be superior to formula. But this benefit is only available if the mother is eating an omega-3 rich diet that allows her to provide her baby with omega-3 fatty acids *in utero* and in her breast milk.

Although omega-3 fatty acids are so important to the growth and development of the fetus/infant, it has been demonstrated that most pregnant and lactating women are often grossly deficient in omega-3—because their diets are devoid of this nutrient. In addition, baby formula manufacturers are currently prohibited from adding omega-3 fatty acids such as DHA to their products. The government has strict guidelines for the manufacture and contents of baby formula; adding DHA would violate these monograph guidelines. Perhaps, in the future, these guidelines will be modified to reflect emerging science. Could it be that this same deficiency of omega-3 fatty acids in the adult diet is linked with congenital or neonatal deficiencies that later manifest as attention deficit disorder?

Another important observation by researchers is that male animals require three times as much essential fatty acids as do females in order to achieve optimal fetal, neonatal, and infant development. This observation in animals is consistent with the human experience that hyperactivity is far more prevalent among boys than among girls.

was reminiscent of the governmental dissemination of the mind-numbing drug Soma in Aldous Huxley's prophetic book *Brave New World*. While this drugging of children seems so egregious for those of us who know better, for the vast majority of these kids, this kind of unnatural pharmaceutical intervention is thought to be absolutely necessary.

Too many parents expect too much from their kids. They put too much pressure on them. If your girl is not Britney Spears or your boy is not worrying about his defined benefit plan, then they're just not with it and you, the parent, take it all personally. That's the way many people (whom we hesitate to call parents) think about their children. If the kids fidget or get bored, it's their fault, too. By God, medicate that child. Fix it quick!

Take the case of Andrea Okeson. She was 13 when she experienced a myriad of symptoms that we used to call teenage anxiety. As reporter Jeffrey Kluger reports in the November 3, 2003 issue of *Time*, "There were the constant stomach pains to consider; there was the nervousness, the distractibility, the overwhelming need to be alone. And, of course, there was the business of repeatedly checking the locks on the doors. All these things grew, inexplicably, to consume Andrea, until by the time she was through with the eighth grade, she seemed pretty much through with everything else too." When the doctors got into the mix, she was basically turned into a mental case. She was diagnosed with generalized anxiety, obsessive-compulsive disorder (OCD) and ADHD.

Today, at 18, she is a student at the College of St. Catherine in St. Paul, Minnesota, and on two types of medication: Lexapro, an antidepressant, and Adderall, an ADHD drug. She tells *Time*: "I feel excited about things. I feel like I got me back."

"Good news all around, right?" asks *Time*. Well, yes—and no. Lexapro is the perfect answer for anxiety all right, provided you're willing to overlook the fact that it does its work by artificially manipulating the very chemicals responsible for feeling and thought. Adderall is the perfect answer for ADHD, given that it's a stimulant like Dexedrine. You also have to overlook the fact that the Adderall has left Andrea with such side effects as weight loss and sleeplessness, and both drugs are being poured into a young brain that has years to go before it's fully formed.

Those things—whether Lexapro or Ritalin or Prozac or something else—are being done for more and more American children. In fact, they are being done with such frequency that some people have justifiably begun to ask, "Are we raising Generation Rx?"

Professor Julie Zito of the University of Maryland School of Pharmacy reports that antidepressant use among children and teens increased by 300 percent in the decade between 1987 and 1996—and is steadily climbing. "Nobody, not even the drug companies, argues that pills alone are the ideal answer to mental illness," She writes. "Most experts believe that drugs are most effective when combined with talk therapy or other counseling.

"Nonetheless, the American Academy of Child and Adolescent Psychiatry now lists dozens of medications available for troubled kids, from the comparatively familiar Ritalin (for ADHD) to Zoloft and Celexa (for depression) to less familiar ones like Seroquel, Tegretol, Depakote (for bipolar disorder), and more are coming along all the time. There are stimulants, mood stabilizers, sleep medications, antidepressants, anticonvulsants, antipsychotics, antianxieties and narrowcast drugs to deal with impulsiveness and post-traumatic flashbacks. A few of the newest meds were developed or approved specifically for kids. The majority have been okayed for adults only, but are being used 'off label' for younger and younger patients at children's menu doses. The practice is common and perfectly legal but potentially risky."

"We know that kids are not just little adults," Dr. David Fassler, professor of psychiatry at the University of Vermont, told *Time*. "They metabolize medications differently."

If we can get our children help through counseling, parental attention and, when needed, natural pathways, this can do a lot more for them than simply medicating. The problem with our quick-fix culture is that if we promise it to parents, they will use and worry about the consequences later. But the brain continues to fully develop until we are in at least our thirties, and we don't know what these profoundly powerful medications will do in the long run to brain development. Will these children be forever medicated? The plain fact is that we're experimenting on these kids.

"Unless there is careful assessment, we might start medicating normal variations (in behavior)," Stephen Hinshaw, chairman of psychology at the University of California, Berkeley, told *Time*.

In May 2000, a Dallas law firm filed a lawsuit against the Swiss drug company Novartis AG, which manufactures Ritalin.[144] The suit seeks class-action status on behalf of people who bought Ritalin for their children. Also named in the suit were the American Psychiatric Association and the advocacy group Children and Adults with Attention-Deficit Hyperactivity Disorder, in Landover, Maryland; both were alleged to have generated concern about the condition while promoting Ritalin and receiving funding from Novartis. Although Novartis has called the lawsuit "without merit" and vowed to "vigorously" defend itself, it is predicted that numerous other suits will soon be filed.

It isn't that drugs such as Ritalin are evil. But, these are, after all, drugs. Doesn't it seem strange—and perhaps even a bit hypocritical—that while America wages its "war against [illegal] drugs" so many children are being placed on drugs that may be legal but also are dangerous to their short- and long-term health? Of course, these drugs help some children. But why are so many kids being medicated? What are the deeper problems that we are failing to deal with?

Ritalin, pemoline (Cylert), dextroamphetamine (Dexedrine) and amphetamine (Adderall) are all stimulants. They are basically legalized "speed." And they do help a number of children, so we can't tell parents to never use them. However, "none of these drugs will cure ADHD," notes Andrew Adesman, M.D.[145]

Still, "when they're effective, they can improve attention, reduce restlessness and foster better relations with peers, parents and teachers," adds Dr. Adesman.

Each of the three stimulants medications has roughly a 75 percent response rate. But when all are used, until one is found to be effective, the response rate is said to be 90 percent.

Still, we do wonder if adding one more drug to childhood is wise. . . .

NOT JUST A DISORDER OF CHILDREN

When the average American thinks of ADHD, she thinks usually of children with behavior problems. This view is understandable because the disorder is so very commonly diagnosed among school-age children, with an incidence ranging from four to 24 percent. But persons with attention difficulties in childhood do not necessarily experience a resolution when they enter adulthood. According to the October 27, 2003 issue of *Business Week,* only three to five percent of children are said to have full-blown ADHD (other sources put the number quite a bit higher), but two-thirds of these children will continue to suffer from the same condition as adults. As Dr. Eugene Arnold, M.D., professor of psychiatry at Ohio State University, states, "ADHD is not just a childhood disorder. A surprising number of adults are affected as well."

American pharmaceutical firms are targeting their ADHD drugs at adults. But if you're an adult with ADHD or symptoms that mirror this condition, we suggest non-toxic nutritional support as your first line of defense.

FYI: One-a-Day Ritalin on the Way

Because children often require multiple doses of these medications, and it is difficult to insure compliance, the drug firm Noven Pharmaceuticals, Inc., of Miami, Florida, is now researching a kids' one-a-day Ritalin, as well as a Ritalin patch.[146]

Meanwhile, Celgene Corp. is working with Novartis to market a highly purified form of Ritalin that is said to be an IQ booster as well. We have reservations (see Ritalin Dangers).

Attention deficit disorder kids are now adults and a whole new marketing push has begun to make sure grown-ups are using drugs too. Take Michael Wendell. The *Business Week* article previously mentioned reports the 32-year-old software engi-

---

Did You Know?
Ritalin Dangers

According to an October 20, 1995 Drug Enforcement Administration bulletin:

- Methylphenidate (MPH), most commonly known as Ritalin, ranks in the top 10 most frequently reported controlled pharmaceuticals stolen from licensed handlers.

- Abuse of MPH can lead to marked tolerance and severe psychic dependence.

- Organized drug trafficking groups in a number of states have utilized various schemes to obtain MPH for resale on the illicit market.

- MPH is abused by diverse segments of the population, from health care professionals and children to street addicts.

- A significant number of children and adolescents are diverting or abusing MPH medication intended for the treatment of ADHD.

- In 1994, a national high school survey (Monitoring the Future) indicated that more seniors in the U.S. abuse Ritalin than are prescribed Ritalin legitimately.

- Students are giving and selling their medication to classmates who are crushing and snorting the powder like cocaine. In March of 1995, two deaths in Mississippi and Virginia were associated with this activity.

- DAWN statistics on estimated emergency room mentions indicate that there were 271 mentions in 1990, 657 mentions in 1991, 1,044 mentions in 1992 and 725 in 1993 (of which 28 to 40 percent were associated with abuse for dependence for psychological effects). The number of mentions for MPH was significantly greater than mentions for Schedule II stimulants (six mentions in 1992 and one mention in 1993 for Schedule III stimulants).

- The U.S. manufactures and consumes five times more MPH than the rest of the world combined.

- MPH aggregate production quota has increased almost sixfold since 1990.

- Ritalin causes cancer.

neer always had problems in school. "He had trouble making friends, couldn't stick to a schedule, and was two to three years behind his classmates in emotional maturity. By third grade, a teacher recommended that he see a therapist, who diagnosed depression."

"But I didn't really fit the typical depressive profile," he tells the news magazine. When Wendell was in his early twenties, he went to a therapist and was diagnosed with attention deficit/hyperactivity disorder (ADHD). "He now takes a cocktail of four drugs every day to keep his symptoms in check," reports *Business Week*.

Such cases help explain why Eli Lilly & Co. has been running a major advertising campaign for the past six months to promote Strattera. The nonstimulant, selective norepinephrine reuptake inhibitor is the first drug the Food and Drug Administration has approved for ADHD in adults. Meanwhile, Shire Pharmaceuticals Group PLC expects to gain FDA approval later this year for its ADHD drug, Adderall XR.

"Both companies see a huge untapped market," says *Business Week*. "Over the past 15 years, mental health specialists have realized that a diagnosis long identified with children also applies from 2 to 4 percent of the adult U.S. population," which is about eight million people. Yet, less than ten percent of these eight million adults now receive treatment. A $2 billion annual market for ADHD pharmaceuticals could double if the drug makers can get more doctors to prescribe such drugs to adult patients.

According to experts cited by the magazine, "These adults tend to change jobs frequently, have substance abuse and gambling problems, commit more crimes, and have a higher divorce rate than the public at large. They often suffer from depression, anxiety, and low self-esteem."

Scientists are currently honing in on two different chemicals found in large amounts in the brain's learning center in the frontal lobes. These include dopamine for maintaining attentiveness and norepinephrine for decision-making.

In the past, children have been treated with stimulants such as Ritalin, Concerta and Adderall. These drugs also raise neurotransmitter levels in the brain but are

Did You Know?
What is ADHD?

Attention-deficit/hyperactivity disorder (ADHD) is a medical term that describes children or adults who are chronically inattentive, uncontrollably impulsive, and hyperactive in a manner inappropriate for mental and chronological age. They often have problems both at home and school. As they grow up they are more likely to drop out of high school and experience patterns of antisocial behavior.

clear-cut stimulants. For adults, the problem with these drugs is that doctors are wary of putting adults on "speed."

But with Strattera, the amount of norepinephrine in the brain can be increased without a stimulant effect. Studies have demonstrated improved organization among adult users. According to the magazine, "Lilly launched Strattera last January and began advertising to consumers in the spring. The ads paid off, with sales of the $3 daily pill totaling $75 million in the second quarter."

ARE HYPERACTIVE CHILDREN AND ADULTS DIFFERENT?

This question has been posed over the last few decades. In order to fully understand its implications, a principle must be understood. Disease arises from a complex interaction of inherent (genetic) susceptibilities and exposure to stressors that trigger innate genetic tendencies to manifest. A New Zealand research group investigated compared 48 hyperactive children to 49 age-and-sex-matched controls to see whether there is indeed a set of characteristics that distinguish children and adults with ADHD from those who do not suffer this malady. Their observations were striking:

- More hyperactive children had auditory, visual, language, reading, and learning difficulties;
- The birth weight of hyperactive children was significantly lower than that of controls;
- More hyperactive children had frequent coughs and colds, and excessive thirst and urination;
- The levels of essential fatty acids were significantly lower in hyperactive children than in the controls.[147]

The therapeutic and diagnostic implications of these findings are intriguing. It seems that hyperactive children are primed for certain difficulties based on a combination of genetic inheritance and environment, including nutritional status.

BRING BACK DR. FEINGOLD

A basic, time-honored principle of naturopathic and homeopathic medicine is to eliminate obstacles to healing. Benjamin F. Feingold, M.D., discovered a modern, direct application of this concept for ADHD. This pioneering pediatrician discovered in the 1960s that the dietary elimination of artificial colorings, flavorings, preservatives, and other artificial food additives reduced hyperactivity in children. His advocacy of the elimination diet to test the applicability of this approach to individual children revolutionized ADHD treatment in the 1970s. Unfortunately, since his death in 1982, a new national leader championing this approach has not emerged. Nevertheless, the validity of this approach as a first therapeutic step continues to be confirmed in clinical practice by professionals progressive enough to try it.

Recent studies confirm what Dr. Feingold uncovered decades ago—that the elimination diet is very helpful in many cases of ADHD.[148,149] Parents and professionals usually find that each child responds to a unique array of chemical additives. And, of course, refined carbohydrates with a high glycemic index (blood sugar raising potential) must also be avoided.

With this backdrop, we can now address the role of fatty acids in ADHD.

HOT ON THE TRAIL OF DISCOVERY

The Hyperactive Children's Support Group (HCSG) is a British organization devoted to helping such children and their families. After conducting surveys of families affected by ADHD and reviewing the scientific literature more than two decades ago, HCSG concluded that many of these children have a deficiency of essential fatty acids either because:

- they cannot metabolize fatty acids normally;
- or they cannot absorb fatty acids efficiently from the gut;
- or their EFA requirements are higher than normal.

To support their conclusions, HCSG points out:

- Most food constituents troublesome in these children are weak inhibitors of the conversion of EFAs to prostaglandins, local tissue hormones.
- Boys are much more commonly affected than girls and have much higher EFA requirements than females.
- Abnormal thirst observed in these children is a sign of EFA deficiency.
- Many ADHD children have eczema, allergies and asthma, which can be alleviated by EFAs. "ADHD children also tend to have more allergies, eczema, asthma, headaches, stomachaches, ear infections and dry skin than non-ADHD youngsters," note researchers Donald Rudin, M.D. and Clara Felix.[150] (Rudin received his medical degree from Harvard Medical School and from 1957 to 1980 served as the director of the Department of Molecular Biology at the Eastern Pennsylvania Psychiatric Institute, Philadelphia. Felix received her B.S. in nutrition from the University of California, Berkeley. Together, they authored *Omega-3 Oils: A Practical Guide.*) Both Rudin and Felix claim ADHD and related disorders are part of a modernization-disease syndrome, which arises from malnutrition centered on an omega-3 fatty acid deficiency.

- Many ADHD children are deficient in zinc, a nutritional cofactor required for conversion of EFAs to prostaglandins.
- Some ADHD children are adversely affected by wheat and milk, known to give rise to exorphin compounds in the gut, which can block conversion of EFAs to beneficial prostaglandin E1.[151]
- The connection between omega-3 fatty acid deficiency and ADHD has been confirmed by studies in which youngsters with ADHD, when compared with non-ADHD children, had much lower blood levels of DHA, the omega-3 fatty acid necessary for normal function of the eyes and the cerebral cortex (the brain region that handles higher functions such as reasoning and memory).

It is astonishing that all this was understood more than twenty years ago by people who were involved in the daily care and nurturance of ADHD children. Yet, to this day, little of this insight is applied in conventional clinical practice.

A Purdue University research group has noted that, according to several studies, some physical symptoms of ADHD are similar to those observed in essential fatty acid deficiency.[152,153] It has been reported that a category of ADHD patients exhibits significantly lower plasma arachidonic acid and docosahexaenoic acid than ADHD persons with few such symptoms or controls. In addition, persons with lower total omega-3 fatty acids have significantly more "behavioral problems, temper tantrums, and learning, health, and sleep problems" than those with high omega-3 fatty acids. The cause of these deficits is unclear. Factors involving fatty acid intake, conversion of essential fatty acids, especially ALA, to EPA and DHA, and enhanced metabolism may be involved. Because the team suspects that DHA is the key to such cases, a study is now proceeding to investigate the effect of oral DHA supplements on the behavior of ADHD children.

HOW OMEGA-3 FATTY ACIDS HELP ADHD CHILDREN:
PROMISING EVIDENCE FOR NUTRITIONAL CURE

You'll want to know about the growing medical evidence that omega-3 fatty acids may also help—without the dangerous complications of Ritalin. There are some key clues as to why non-drug remedies may be even more effective.

All cells throughout the human body are enveloped by membranes composed chiefly of essential fatty acids in the form of phospholipids. Phospholipids play a major role in determining the integrity and fluidity of cell membranes. What determines the type of phospholipid in the cell membrane is the type of fat consumed. Unfortunately, our children's diets, which may be laden with saturated and unfavorable polyunsaturated fats from beef, dairy, and corn oil, interfere with the optimal balance of phospholipids in cell membranes. When the cell membranes are composed of saturated fats or omega-6 fatty acids, children may exhibit all of the symptoms of ADHD.

A phospholipid composed of a saturated fat or trans-fatty acid differs considerably in structure from a phospholipid composed of an essential fatty acid. In addition, there are differences between the structure of an omega-3 oil-composed membrane and an omega-6 composed membrane. Up to 80 percent of the fatty acids in the cerebral cortex of the brain should be composed of omega-3 fatty acids. (Food sources particularly rich in omega-3 fatty acids include cold-water fish and flaxseed oil.)

It is thought that the cell is programmed to selectively incorporate the different fatty acids it needs to maintain optimal function, assuming that what the cell needs is in adequate supply from the diet. In actuality, what becomes incorporated into the cell membranes is determined primarily by diet. A diet composed of largely saturated fat, cholesterol, and trans-fatty acids, such as the junk food American diet, is going to lead to membranes which are much less fluid and much more dysfunctional in nature compared to the membranes of an individual consuming optimal levels of essential fatty acids. Children with such imbalances are more likely to display aggressive, impulsive, and disruptive behavior, lack desirable attention spans, and are more likely to exhibit antisocial behavior.

"A relative deficiency of essential fatty acids in cellular membranes makes it virtually impossible for the cell membrane to perform its vital functions," says noted naturopathic physician Michael Murray, N.D.:

> The basic function of the cell membrane is to serve as a selective barrier that regulates the passage of certain materials in and out of the cell. When there is a disturbance of structure or function of the cell membrane, there is a tremendous disruption of homeostasis. This term, homeostasis, refers to the maintenance of static conditions in the internal environment of the cell and, on a larger scale, the human body as a whole. In other words, with a disturbance in cellular membrane structure or function, there is a disruption of virtually all cellular processes.

Because the brain is the richest repository of phospholipids in the human body, and accurate nerve cell function is critically dependent on proper membrane fluidity and integrity, it only makes sense that alterations in membrane fluidity could dramatically impact behavior, mood, and mental function, adds Dr. Murray. In addition, studies have shown that biophysical properties, including fluidity of

synaptic membranes, directly influences neurotransmitter synthesis, signal trans-
duction, uptake of serotonin and other neurotransmitters, and neurotransmitter
binding. All of these factors have been implicated in depression and other psychological disturbances in children.

SCIENTIFIC EVIDENCE

Two types of fatty acids are considered essential. Omega-3 and omega-6 fatty
acids cannot be synthesized in the body, and must be obtained from the diet.
Furthermore, omega-3 fatty acids cannot be converted to omega-6 fats and vice
versa. What you eat is what you get. The omega-6 fatty acids are distributed evenly
in most tissues and easily obtained through food sources commonly found in the
American diet. But omega-3 fatty acids are concentrated in a few tissues including
the brain.[154,155] Because of their relative scarcity in the American diet, many children—
perhaps a majority of children today—are deficient in omega-3 fatty acids. Learning
specialists now believe omega-3 fatty acid deficiency leads to unique symptoms during childhood, including behavioral problems.[156,157]

The evidence is certainly suggestive. In 1981, researchers first hypothesized that
children with ADHD may have reduced nutritional status of essential fatty acids
because they showed greater thirst (a symptom of essential fatty acid deficiency)
compared to children without ADHD.[158] These results were further confirmed in a
1983 study involving 23 maladjusted children and 20 normal children; essential
fatty acid blood levels in poorly behaved children were significantly lower.[159]

In 1987, researchers further documented the link between symptoms of an essential fatty acid deficiency and behavioral problems. When they looked at 48 children
with ADHD, there was significantly greater thirst, more frequent urination, and more
health and learning problems than in children without ADHD.[160] Significantly lower
levels of two omega-6 fatty acids and one omega-3 fatty acid (DHA) were found in
the subjects with ADHD symptoms.

In a 1995 study comparing plasma essential fatty acid levels in 53 boys with
ADHD to a control group of 43 boys without ADHD, researchers found significantly
lower levels of omega-3 fatty acids.[161]

In the April-May 1996 issue of *Physiology & Behavior,* Laura J. Stevens of the
Department of Foods and Nutrition, Purdue University and co-investigators found that
boys with lower levels of omega-3 fatty acids in their blood showed more problems with
behavior, learning, and health than those with higher levels of total omega-3 fatty
acids.[162] That same year, researchers from the Department of Psychiatry and Faculty of
Medicine at Technical University in Trabzon, Turkey reported that levels of free fatty

acids, as well as zinc, were severalfold lower in ADHD children compared to non-ADHD children.[163] Zinc is a known cofactor for the proper metabolism of essential fatty acids.

Most recently, researchers performed a study to test the effect of omega-3 fatty acids on intelligence scores among 56 18-month-old children.[164] The children were divided into three groups: one received DHA, the second received DHA and arachidonic acid, and the third a formula that did not contain either. All children were enrolled in the study within five days of birth and received one of the three formulas for 17 weeks. The children's overall intelligence and motor skills were tested using the latest Bayley Scales of Infant Development (BSID), the standard for gauging the development of small children. No differences were seen in the Psychomotor Development Index. On the Mental Development Index, which measures memory, ability to solve simple problems and language capabilities, the children in the control group received an average score of 98, slightly below the national average of 100. The DHA group received an average score of 102.4 and the DHA and arachidonic acid group received an average score of 105.1. The children will be tested again in four years to see if the gains continue into early childhood.

OPTIMIZING RESULTS

There are no magic bullets in natural medicine. Because essential fatty acids are building blocks for every cell membrane in the body, their wide-ranging effects make them seem like panaceas. Nevertheless, it is imperative for parents and medical professionals to be aware of dosing considerations and synergistic items that can optimize clinical outcomes.

According to research in cardiovascular disease, arthritis, and inflammatory bowel disease, the effective adult dosage range for EPA and DHA is three to five grams daily in divided doses. This dosage can be adjusted downward in proportion to body weight to meet the needs of children. In addition, sufficient time must be allowed for the fatty acids to become incorporated into cell membranes and other tissues. Turnover of fatty acids on cell membranes takes time, especially among children whose bodies have been starving for good fatty acid nutrition since conception. It takes at least six months, in some cases, to see gratifying results.

A broad-range high-potency, hypoallergenic vitamin and mineral supplement is indicated to correct micronutrient deficiencies noted in these patients. For children, zinc is particularly important (with a small amount of counter-balancing copper) due to its identification as a nutrient specifically lacking in ADHD children.

In order to maximize the beneficial effects of omega-3 nutrition, apply the Feingold dietary ideas to remove the adverse effects of artificial additives and refined

Fish Oils May Help Dyslexic Children

According to the International Health News Database...

GUILDFORD, UNITED KINGDOM. Dyslexia is a fairly common condition that involves difficulties in learning to read and write, mirror reversals of letters and words, and poor short-term memory. Dyslexia is closely related to dyspraxia (problems with coordination and muscle control) and attention-deficit hyperactivity disorder. It is estimated that about 10 percent of the populations of the United States and the United Kingdom suffer from dyslexia and four percent are severely affected. There was a three-fold increase in the prevalence of learning disorders in the United States over the period 1976 to 1993 and 80 percent of the new cases involved dyslexia.

Dr. Jacqueline Stordy of the University of Surrey believes that dyslexia, dyspraxia, and attention-deficit hyperactivity disorder have one common denominator—a deficiency of long-chain fatty acids.[165] She points to a study that found improved dark adaptation (the adjustment of the eyes to the dark, a problem among dyslexics) after supplementation with 480 mg a day of docosahexaenoic acid (a main constituent of fish oil) for a month. Another study involving fifteen dyspractic children found that supplementation with a proprietary mixture of tuna oil, evening primrose oil, thyme oil, and vitamin E for four months markedly improved their motor skills. The mixture provided 480 mg of docosahexaenoic acid, 35 mg of arachidonic acid, 96 mg of alpha-linolenic acid, 80 mg of vitamin E, and 24 mg of thyme oil daily. Dr. Stordy concludes that long-chain polyunsaturated fatty acid supplements may benefit children with dyslexia, dyspraxia, and attention-deficit hyperactivity disorder and notes that large, double-blind, placebo-controlled studies are already underway to verify this hypothesis.

carbohydrates, and foods to which the child is sensitive. The removal of these obstacles to healing takes avoidable and undesirable stress off the child's metabolic processes. This is crucial information, especially for parents of children who are diagnosed with ADHD and who are presently being prescribed Ritalin.

"We shouldn't be prescribing medicine simply because that's the easiest way to go," notes Dr. Mark Stein, who runs a University of Chicago clinic for children and adults with the disorder. While all children with ADHD are not deficient in omega-3 fatty acids, we believe that this may be important for at least a major subset of ADHD children. And omega-3 fatty acids may make a dramatic difference among these children. If your ADHD child is not among these, the omega-3 fatty acids nevertheless have many other benefits.

In fact, studies show that children whose treatment program includes only medication, educational and psychological therapy continue to be at high risk for vandalism, petty crime, frequency of alcoholic intoxication, and possession of marijuana. Dietary improvements may be the key to fostering long-term mental health and acceptable behavior.

Parents of ADHD children and ADHD adults who wish to utilize omega-3 fatty acids as a method of modifying their behavior should use pure fish oil and wild ocean fish, which are the best way to go. Avoid fried food sources of trans fatty acids that inactivate conversion enzymes and ensure an adequate intake of vitamins B_3, B_6, and C, zinc, and magnesium to support enzyme activity. Wild fish or pure fish oil capsules provide DHA directly, which appears to be a vital omega-3 fatty acid for modifying the behavior of ADHD children and adults.

A combination of flax seed and wild fish is best, especially since flax can be so easily incorporated into baked foods, salad dressings, and even delicious types of deserts.

Nursing mothers may have even lower levels of essential fatty acids unless they supplement. We recommend that pregnant and nursing women take one to two pure fish oil capsules daily that are guaranteed by laboratory analysis to be free from toxic pollutants.

CHAPTER 5

Omega-3s &
Pregnancy Outcome

All over the world, excellent studies document the need for omega-3s and show us that fish consumption during pregnancy is generally safe, although we think all women of childbearing age should be prudent and avoid contaminated seafood whenever possible. Let's take a little adventure—via the International Health Database....

HEALTHY BABIES AND FISH CONSUMPTION

COPENHAGEN, DENMARK. Danish researchers report that women who consume fish or seafood once a week during the first 16 weeks of pregnancy have 3.6 times a lower risk of giving birth to a low birth weight (less than 2,500 grams) or a premature (born before 259 days) baby than do women who never consume fish or seafood. The study involved almost 9,000 women who completed a food frequency questionnaire. The researchers found that women whose daily intake of fish was less than 15 grams, corresponding to a fish oil intake of 150 mg/day, were significantly more likely to give birth to a preterm or underweight baby than were women with higher intakes. They suggest that small amounts of fish oil may confer protection against preterm delivery and low birth weight.[166]

MATERNAL MILK AND DHA SUPPLEMENTATION

MUNICH, GERMANY. DHA is vital for the proper development of an infant's brain and retina. DHA must be supplied through mother's milk or infant formula, as the infant itself is unable to synthesize it from other dietary sources such as flax oil. The DHA content of human milk varies from 0.05 percent in vegetarian women to 1.40 percent in Inuit women. An average level in omnivorous women is about 0.3 percent by weight. It is assumed that a mother's diet affects the composition of her breast milk, but no specific studies of the transfer of DHA to breast milk has been made so far. Researchers at the Ludwig-Maximilian-Universitat now report that an increased dietary intake of DHA by a lactating woman results in a proportional increase in her breast milk. Their study involved 10 lactating women who between four and six weeks in the postpartum stage supplemented with either 200 mg of DHA per day or 200 mg of a corn/soy oil mixture (placebo oil). At the end of the two weeks the DHA content of the milk from the DHA-supplemented mothers had increased by 28 percent while the DHA content in the milk from the mothers in the placebo group had decreased by 25 percent. In other words, after two weeks the DHA content in the milk from DHA-supplemented mothers was almost twice as high as in the milk from the mothers in the placebo group. There were no significant differences in the amount of milk produced per day by the 2 groups. (Editor's note: Supplementation with DHA would be particularly important for lactating mothers who are vegetarian.)[167]

FISH OIL SUPPLEMENTATION DURING PREGNANCY IS SAFE

ADELAIDE, AUSTRALIA. There is still considerable controversy regarding the role of long chain omega-3 polyunsaturated fatty acids (PUFAs) in infant development and little attention has been paid to the requirements of mothers for these nutrients. Two researchers at the University of Adelaide have just released a review of existing research findings concerning these subjects. One clinical trial found that women who supplemented with fish oil (1.5 grams eicosapentaenoic acid [EPA] and one gram docosahexaenoic acid [DHA] daily) from their 30th week of pregnancy extended the pregnancy by four days and gave birth to infants weighing an average of 100 grams more that infants born to mothers supplementing with placebos (olive oil). Other studies have failed to confirm these effects.

A recent study found that DHA levels decrease rapidly in women after giving birth independent of whether they are breastfeeding or not. There is speculation that this relative DHA deficiency could be a major factor in postpartum depression, but clinical trials are needed to confirm this. The deficiency can be completely eliminated by supplementing with 200 to 400 mg/day of DHA. The evidence concerning the benefits of maternal DHA supplementation on infant development is inconclusive.

One study found that infants with an adequate DHA status at three months of age scored better on a mental development test at age one year, but not at two years of age. The researchers conclude that there is no evidence that maternal DHA supplementation is harmful and that it may have subtle benefits to both mother and infant. However, further clinical trials are needed to verify this.[168]

FORMULA-FED INFANTS NEED DHA

TORONTO, CANADA. A team of researchers from Canada, Britain, and the United States emphasize the importance of ensuring that newborn infants get sufficient DHA in order to ensure optimal neural and visual development during the first six months of life. They point out that there is still controversy as to whether the required DHA can be synthesized by the infants themselves (from alpha-linolenic acid) or must be supplied by the diet—be it breast milk or infant formula. The researchers reviewed numerous studies comparing the DHA status of breast-fed infants with that of formula-fed ones. They found that over the first six months of life DHA accumulates in the body of breast-fed infants at a rate of 10 mg/day with 48 percent of this accumulation occurring in the brain. They estimate that an intake of 20 mg/day of DHA is required to achieve this accumulation and point out that breastfeeding supplies about 60 mg/day. They believe the seeming over-abundance of DHA in breast milk may be needed in order to provide for potentially increased losses during disease, infection, surgery, and other conditions adversely affecting the infants' metabolism.

On the other hand, formula-fed infants would seem to develop a serious deficiency of DHA if they are fed a formula not fortified with DHA (usually in combination with arachidonic acid). Standard infant formulas contribute about 390 mg/day of alpha-linolenic acid so about 5.2 percent of this would have to be converted to DHA in order to produce the needed 20 mg/day. The researchers point out that there is no evidence at all that infants are able to achieve this conversion rate and speculate that the rate may be as much as 20 times lower than required. This conclusion is amply supported by the fact that formula-fed infants actually lose 993 mg of DHA over the first six months of life, while breast-fed babies gain an average of 1,882 mg. The accumulation of DHA in the brain of formula-fed infants is only half of that observed in breast-fed infants and while the liver in breast-fed infants gains 24 mg of DHA during the first six months the liver in formula-fed ones actually loses 136 mg.

The researchers conclude that feeding infants with a non-fortified formula will not provide the DHA provided by breast milk. They urge further work to determine whether a formula containing at least 0.2 percent DHA (providing 60 mg/day of DHA) will provide equivalent DHA accumulation to that of breast-fed infants.[169]

DHA FORTIFIES BREAST MILK

HOUSTON, TEXAS. Docosahexaenoic acid is an important component of brain cell membranes; a deficiency during infancy has been linked to poorer brain development and a decline in visual acuity. DHA occurs naturally in breast milk, but is absent in most infant formulas. Surveys have shown that the DHA content in breast milk from American women tends to be lower than that in milk from women in most other countries.

Researchers at the Baylor College of Medicine now report that the DHA content of breast milk can be increased by supplementing with DHA and that this higher DHA content is transferred to breast-fed infants.[170] The study involved 26 pregnant women who planned to breast feed exclusively for at least eight weeks after giving birth. The women were randomly assigned to one of four groups and given either a daily DHA supplement or a placebo from two weeks after giving birth to eight weeks after giving birth. Group 1 received an algae-produced triacylglycerol with a high DHA content (providing less than 230 mg/day of DHA); Group 2 consumed two high DHA content eggs (providing 170 mg/day of DHA); Group 3 took a low EPA, high DHA fish oil (providing 260 mg/day of DHA); and Group 4 (the control group) consumed two regular eggs daily (providing less than 35 mg/day of DHA).

All three forms of DHA supplements produced significant increases in the DHA content of the women's blood plasma (phospholipid phase) and breast milk. Consumption of two eggs per day over a six-week period was well tolerated by all participants and had no adverse effects on cholesterol or triglyceride levels. The DHA level in the blood plasma (phospholipid phase) of the breast-fed infants also increased significantly over the six-week supplementation period with the infants in groups 1 and 3 having the largest increases.

INFANTS NEED LONG-CHAIN OMEGA-3 FATTY ACIDS

KANSAS CITY, MISSOURI. It is well established that human infants require an adequate supply of omega-3 and omega-6 long-chain polyunsaturated fatty acids for optimal growth and neural development. There is evidence that the need for omega-3 acids, particularly DHA, is especially pronounced among pre-term infants. It has been suggested that these infants lack the ability to synthesize DHA from alpha-linolenic acid in sufficient amounts to ensure an adequate supply to the brain and retina. Several studies have shown that pre-term infants fed a formula with added DHA developed better visual acuity and retinal response to light and scored higher when evaluated for mental development. Among in-term infants fed a DHA-fortified formula, some studies, but not all, have found higher visual acuity and better problem-solving ability. Dr. S.E. Carlson of the University of Missouri supports the idea of adding DHA to infant formulas, but cautions that his fortification should be balanced with an appropriate addition of long-chain omega-6 acids (arachidonic acid) in order to more closely approximate the composition of mother's milk.[171]

YOUR BRAIN NEEDS DHA

NEW YORK, NEW YORK. Dr. Barbara Levine, Professor of Nutrition in Medicine at Cornell University, sounds the alarm concerning a totally inadequate intake of DHA by most Americans.[172] DHA is the building block of human brain tissue and is particularly abundant in the gray matter of the brain and the retina. Low levels of DHA have recently been associated with depression, memory loss, dementia, and visual problems. DHA is particularly important for fetuses and infants; the DHA content of the infant's brain triples during the first three months of life. Optimal levels of DHA are therefore crucial for pregnant and lactating mothers.

Unfortunately, the average DHA content of breast milk in the United States is the lowest in the world, most likely because Americans eat comparatively little fish. Making matters worse is the fact that the United States is the only country in the world where infant formulas are not fortified with DHA—despite a 1995 recommendation by the World Health Organization that all baby formulas should provide 40 mg of DHA per kilogram of infant body weight. Dr. Levine believes that postpartum depression, attention-deficit/hyperactivity disorder (ADHD), and low IQs are all linked to the dismally low DHA intake common in the United States. Dr. Levine also points out that low DHA levels have been linked to low brain serotonin levels, which again are connected to an increased tendency towards depression, suicide, and violence. DHA is abundant in marine phytoplankton and cold-water fish, and nutritionists now recommend that people consume two to three servings of fish every week to maintain DHA levels. If this is not possible, Dr. Levine suggests supplementing with 100 mg of DHA a day.

MOTHERS' FISH OIL
SUPPLEMENTATION BENEFITS INFANTS

PORTLAND, OREGON. Animal experiments have shown that monkeys born by mothers with low blood levels of docosahexaenoic acid (DHA) develop impaired vision. There is also evidence that premature human infants fed standard infant formulas (very low in DHA) have impaired visual function, which can be improved significantly by adding fish oils to their formulas. All this adds to the growing evidence that DHA is essential for the proper development of the brain and retina in the fetus and infant. Researchers at the Oregon Health Sciences University recently set out to answer the question, "Do high intakes of DHA by pregnant women increase the DHA level in their newborn infants?"[173] Their clinical trial involved 31 healthy, pregnant women, 15 of whom were assigned to receive 2.6 grams/day of omega-3 fatty acid from fish (1.01 grams DHA/day) from their 26th to their 35th week of pregnancy. The remaining women served as controls. The fish oil supplement was taken as a varying combination of tinned sardines and fish oil capsules—either one half tin of sardines plus seven fish oil capsules per day, one tin of sardines (3.75 oz) plus three fish oil capsules per day, or ten fish oil capsules (10 g) per day. Blood samples were collected from mothers at entry to the study, monthly after entry and at delivery, and from the infants at delivery. The level of DHA in the red blood cells of supplemented mothers rose from 4.69 percent (of total fatty acids) at entry to 7.15 percent at the end of week 34, and then declined (as expected) to 5.97 percent at delivery. DHA increases in the blood plasma paralleled the increase in the red blood cells, but at a lower level. DHA levels in newborn infants differed greatly depending on whether the mothers had supplemented or not. Red blood cell levels in infants born by supplementing mothers were 35.2 percent higher than in the control infants and blood plasma levels were 45.5 percent higher (5.05 percent vs. 3.47 percent).

The researchers believe that supplementing pregnant mothers with fish oil may benefit brain and retinal development in their offspring particularly if born prematurely. They point out that supplementing from mid-pregnancy to the 34th week is perfectly safe and may reduce the incidence of preeclampsia (pregnancy-related high blood pressure) as well.

DHA HELPS BRAIN DEVELOPMENT

MILAN, ITALY. Researchers at the University of Milan report that infants whose formula contains long-chain polyunsaturated fatty acids (especially DHA) have better brain development than children who do not receive DHA in their formula.[174] The observation supports earlier findings that there is a direct correlation between the DHA concentration in the red blood cells of infants and their visual acuity. The researchers recommend that infants who are not breast-fed be fed on a DHA-enriched formula. Breast milk already contains the fatty acids necessary for good brain development.

CHAPTER 6

Diabetics & Omega-3s

D iabetes mellitus is a chronic disorder involving carbohydrates, fat, and protein metabolism, and characterized by highly increased levels of sugar in the blood, and subsequently, in the urine. In fact, in ancient times, the urine of diabetic patients was described as tasting like honey, sticky to the touch, and strongly attracting ants. In diabetes, either the pancreas fails to secrete adequate amounts of insulin, a hormone produced by the beta cells of the islets of Langerhans in the pancreas that enables sugar to be absorbed by the body's cells, or the body cells become unresponsive or resistant to insulin. When blood sugar cannot enter cells and instead is left in the blood, this causes the complications associated with diabetes including increased risk for heart and circulatory disease, stroke, kidney malfunction, blindness, and loss of nerve function.

"SYNDROME X" AFFLICTS MANY AMERICANS

"Syndrome X" is the name that has been applied by both medical doctors and natural medicine practitioners and researchers to a constellation of symptoms that portend the full onset of adult type II diabetes. The main signs of Syndrome X include high levels of insulin in the blood, obesity, elevated cholesterol and triglycerides, high blood pressure, and tissue insulin resistance.

There is a group of symptoms and signs that is quite indicative of diabetes mellitus. Persons with diabetes urinate much more than normal. Such excessive loss of fluids and high concentration of sugar in the blood cause people to become very thirsty. When people drink sugar-sweetened beverages, they urinate even more and become even more thirsty.

In simple terms, the main job of insulin in the human body is to regulate blood glucose or "blood sugar." It also facilitates the entry of amino acids into the cell. This function is truly critical. If blood glucose rises too high, a person becomes at risk for dehydration, coma, and possibly death. Because the cells (especially neurons in the central nervous system that depend on sugar to function) are internally deprived of glucose tiredness and weakness, accompanied by apathy, are often found in persons with diabetes. People may not be able to even get up in the morning. Tingling may occur in the hands or feet (diabetic neuropathy). There may be reduced resistance to infections such as boils, urinary tract disorders and vaginal fungal infections because the excess blood sugar interferes with the white blood cell utilization of vitamin C.

TWO TYPES OF DIABETES

There are two types of diabetes mellitus. Type I (juvenile-onset) diabetes is also known as insulin-dependent diabetes mellitus (IDDM) and usually arises in children as a result of the destruction of the insulin-producing pancreatic beta cells by the immune system. Type II (adult-onset) diabetes is also known as non-insulin dependent diabetes mellitus (NIDDM). It usually afflicts people past the age of 40. However, due to the rise in obesity in children, there has been an alarming manifestation of Type II diabetes in juveniles. Whereas symptoms may occur within weeks or months in Type I diabetes, symptoms may occur only gradually, long after the disease has set in, in people with Type II diabetes. Only about 10 percent of diabetics are Type I.

Type I diabetes is generally associated with damage to the beta-cells of the pancreas, thus causing people to require lifelong insulin for the control of their blood sugar levels. This damage may be caused by an autoimmune disorder in which the immune system attacks the body's pancreas. In fact, we now know that about 75 percent of cases of Type I diabetes are accompanied by the presence of beta-cell antibodies, which are produced by the immune system to mistakenly attack the pancreatic tissues. (Among persons without Type I diabetes, only about 0.5 to 2 percent of the population have beta-cell antibodies.) However, in non-insulin dependent diabetes, the problem is generally that the body's cells have lost their sensitivity to insulin; we find that too often obesity is a prime contributing factor of loss of sensitivity.

For both types I and II, dietary and nutritional considerations are critical. In fact, for Type II diabetics, diet, nutrition, and exercise are the major initial pathways by which a healing response may be initiated within the body.

Clearly, frequency of diabetes is closely associated with diets lacking adequate fiber and containing excessively refined carbohydrates such as refined sugar.[174] Diets that are rich in legumes (beans) and vegetables are especially helpful, both for better sugar control and weight loss.

INSULIN RESISTANCE: MAJOR FEATURE OF DIABETES

Anyone who is diabetic, or lives with someone who is, knows that one of the main problems in diabetes, especially in the most common occurrence of Type II diabetes known as adult-onset, is *insulin resistance,* and that obesity often accompanies the condition.

After a meal, the rise in blood sugar prompts the pancreas to release insulin into the bloodstream, which causes muscle and fat cells to take up the excess sugar and either use it as fuel or store it in a slightly altered form called glycogen in muscle and as fat in fat cells. When blood sugar levels fall, the pancreas produces another hormone called glucagon that prompts the body to convert the glycogen back into glucose or to form glucose from amino acids.

In a perfect world, this balance between the two hormones—insulin and glucagon—enables the body to maintain blood sugar at optimal levels. Unfortunately, for some 16 million Americans, their body does not respond adequately to insulin and is unable to maintain optimal blood sugar levels.

As a result of insulin resistance, not only do blood sugar levels build-up in the blood, the body also produces excessive amounts of insulin. This combination causes diabetic symptoms such as excessive thirst, frequent urination, fatigue, tingling or burning in the fingers and toes, accelerated cardiovascular damage, diabetic retinopathy, and kidney damage. In addition, continuous high levels of glucose can cause an unfavorable, non-enzyme-driven binding of sugar molecules to protein molecules that can have deleterious effects. If glucose is bound to antigens (identification proteins) on the surface of cell membranes, this restructuring of antigens can be very confusing to the immune system, which relies on antigens to distinguish self from non-self. Depending on the nature of the new, inappropriate protein-sugar complex, the immune system can misread antigens, causing it to attack misidentified healthy cells as foreign invaders or to misread antigens on cancer cells as normal.

MANY AMERICANS AT RISK FOR SYNDROME X

What's more, many Americans, even if not overtly diabetic, are nevertheless insulin resistant and therefore prone to Syndrome X. Indeed, virtually everyone who is overweight or suffers high blood pressure also suffers insulin resistance, says Dr. Artemis Simopoulos, author of *The Omega Diet* (HarperCollins, 1999). She estimates, "as many as half of the adults in this country may suffer from some degree of insulin resistance." Thus, persons suffering obesity and elevated cholesterol or blood pressure can also benefit by emphasizing foods rich in omega-3 fatty acids.

EVIDENCE SUPPORTS ROLE FOR OMEGA-3 FATTY ACIDS

Now there is real hope that a special class of fats, found in a few select foods, can help. Recent new evidence suggests that omega-3 fatty acids like those found in fish oils can have an extremely positive influence on the health of diabetics and the prevention of Syndrome X.

In the modern American diet, healthy omega-3 fatty acids are supplanted by a far greater intake of the omega-6 fatty acids prevalent in most vegetable oils and in saturated fat from commercial beef, pork, dairy, and fried foods.

An interesting Swedish study was published in 1994 reporting the effect of fatty acid nutrition on the development of Type II diabetes.[176] A group of 1,828 men aged 50 were followed for a period of ten years. During that time 75 developed NIDDM. The serum lipid profiles of study participants indicated that, relative to those who did not develop diabetes, those who did had higher saturated fat and omega-6 fatty acids with low amounts of alpha-linolenic acid (ALA). The researchers concluded that Type II diabetes is predictable by the high levels of serum omega-6 fatty acids.

A report from the *Annals of the New York Academy of Sciences* shows that experimental diets high in omega-6 fatty acids produce insulin resistance. However, supplementing with omega-3 fatty acids restores insulin sensitivity—even though the diet remains high in other fats.[177]

Another study shows diets rich in omega-6 fatty acids from soybean or safflower oil or saturated fat induce far greater weight gain than diets that emphasize omega-3 fatty acids.[178] Indeed, in this study, all groups consumed equivalent calories and grams of fat, but the difference between a soybean-oil diet and one rich in omega-3 fatty acids was the difference in weight between a 225- and a 150-pound man.

To determine the effects of fish oil supplementation on lipid levels and glycemic control in patients with Type II diabetes, the Mayo Clinic conducted a recent analysis of all randomized, placebo-controlled trials in which fish oil was the only intervention in subjects with type II diabetes.[179] There were a total of 18 trials including 823 subjects who were followed for an average of 12 weeks. Doses of fish oil used ranged from three to eighteen grams daily. The team found that fish oil consistently lowered triglycerides but raised LDLs. No significant effect was observed for fasting glucose, glucose-bound hemoglobin, total cholesterol, or HDL. The triglyceride lowering and elevation in LDL were most marked in trials with high triglyceride subjects and used higher doses of fish oil.

Unfortunately, these short-term trials may not tell the whole story of what fish oils can do for diabetics. It takes time for membrane fatty acids to turn over sufficiently to achieve their full therapeutic benefits.

An Italian research team noted clear evidence of a significant triglyceride reduction resulting from omega-3 supplements, based on their examination of large population studies that evaluated the development of glucose intolerance or diabetes in patients with predisposing conditions. Long-term supplementation reduced LDL cholesterol, with positive effects on HDL. These are considered constructive changes indicative of improved glucose management. The added cardiovascular benefits of omega-3 fatty acids provide further indication for the use of fish oils in diabetic patients.[180] This analysis reveals the long-term healing potential of fish oils.

The effect of fish oil in preventing diabetic neuropathy has been less impressive than omega-6 fatty acids. This partial effect of omega-3s might be attributed to the presence of EPA, a membrane competitor of omega-6 arachidonic acid. A French team recently conducted an experiment to determine whether supplementing with DHA alone could prevent neuropathy in rats with experimentally induced diabetes.[181] Eight weeks of diabetes induced significant decreases in nerve conduction velocity and nerve blood flow. However, DHA totally prevented the decrease in nerve conduction velocity and nerve blood flow observed during diabetes, when compared with the non-supplemented diabetic group. Moreover, DHA levels in the sciatic nerve membranes (in the lower spinal cord) were correlated with nerve conduction velocity. These results demonstrate a protective effect of DHA on experimental diabetic neuropathy. Based on the findings, the French team suggested a thorough clinical investigation.

PROFOUND HUMAN CONSEQUENCES

Insulin is required for the synthesis of the long-chain omega-3 fatty acids from ALA. Under these conditions, diabetics are left in a state of deficiency in EPA and DHA. As we have discussed in the chapter on cardiovascular disease, this kind of deficiency predisposes diabetics to cardiovascular difficulties, in addition to the vascular problems caused by high blood sugar. Thus, supplementation with the longer chain omega-3 fatty acids found in fish oils is indicated.

In Australia, researcher Leonard A. Storlien discovered that people with muscle cells low in omega-3 fatty acids and high levels of omega-6 fatty acids were most likely to be both insulin-resistant and obese.[182] As the imbalance became more magnified, so did their weight and metabolic problems.

There is hope that dietary changes can enhance the body's insulin sensitivity and reduce the risk for Syndrome X complications. In 1997, 55 persons diagnosed with

Syndrome X were assigned to a diet high in omega-3 fatty acids, particularly fish.[183] After one year, their insulin sensitivity had improved. They also lost weight, and their blood pressure and triglyceride levels decreased.

A second study of 48 people assigned to either a low-calorie but high-carbohydrate diet or a diet rich in omega-3 fatty acids found dramatic health differences between the two groups. After one year, those consuming low-fat high, carbohydrate diets had higher glucose levels and reduced insulin sensitivity.[184] Persons consuming the omega-3 fatty acid-rich diet had enhanced insulin sensitivity with lower blood sugar levels, elevated HDLs (the"good" cholesterol), lower triglycerides, and blood pressure. They had significantly reversed Syndrome X. As Dr. Simopoulos notes, "When your diet contains a healthy ratio of fatty acids, you have a more normal metabolism and a lower risk of Syndrome X, obesity, and diabetes."

HOW TO ENHANCE INSULIN SENSITIVITY

Seek out the advice of a skilled holistic health professional who well understands the causes and natural interventions for Syndrome X. The key to enhancing insulin sensitivity and curbing problems related to Syndrome X is to consume a diet low in simple, refined carbohydrates (such as those found in sweets, desserts, processed baked and prepared foods) and rich in omega-3 fatty acids. You'll want to emphasize wild ocean fish, green leafy vegetables, flax oil, legumes, whole grains and nuts such as walnuts. Appropriate nutritional supplements, including chromium and niacin, are also important. Exercise is vital.

FYI: Typical Foods with Low Glycemic Index

These foods release sugar into the bloodstream gradually and help persons with diabetes or insulin resistance to stabilize their blood sugar levels:

- Legumes (lentils, chick peas, split peas, kidney beans, white beans)
- Whole-grain rye bread
- Whole-grain, high-fiber cereals
- Whole-grain pasta
- Oranges
- Organic milk and yogurt
- Brown Rice
- Bulgar

THE DOCTORS' PRESCRIPTION

Most everyone—particularly persons with diabetes—will benefit from consuming more wild ocean fish such as salmon and fresh tuna, as well as taking one to two capsules of fish oil daily.

FYI: Typical Foods with High Glycemic Index

These foods release large amounts of sugar into the blood stream very quickly and produce sharp rises in blood sugar levels:

- Soft drinks sweetened with sugar
- White rice
- White bread
- Instant mashed potatoes
- Jams and jellies
- High-sugar cereals
- Corn flakes
- Simple sugars
- Corn chips

CHAPTER 7

Female Health:
Omega-3s to the Rescue

PREMENSTRUAL SYNDROME

Premenstrual syndrome (PMS) can affect any woman of menstruating age. One woman in three regularly experience PMS symptoms. One woman in 20 experiences severe psychological and physical symptoms of premenstrual dysphoric disorder (PMDD). Both PMS and PMDD adversely affect a significant proportion of relationships. Both describe a complex group of psychological, behavioral and physical symptoms that affect women in the luteal phase of their menstrual cycle. The luteal phase is the 13th to 14th interlude between ovulation and the onset of the next period. Either PMS or PMDD can affect any woman of menstruating age. Symptoms occur only in the luteal phase of the menstrual cycle and cease at, or soon after, the period—menses—begins.

Why do some women suffer so much menstrual pain? The risk of PMS increases with major hormonal events such as puberty, pregnancy, or childbirth; the use of oral contraception; a hysterectomy; and major stress. Part of the problem might also be a fatty acid imbalance. Prostaglandins are the local hormones made by tissue enzymes using the fatty acids on cell membranes as raw materials. If we eat too many omega-6 fatty acids, we will have an over-abundance of the omega-6 arachidonic acid on the membranes. The local hormones will convert archidonic acid into the kind of prostaglandins that promote muscle constriction. This cramping effect affects the smooth muscle of the uterus.

A Danish research group tested whether menstrual discomfort, known to be prostaglandin-mediated, can be influenced by the dietary ratio of omega-3 to omega-6 fatty acids. A survey using a self-administered questionnaire concerning menstrual history, present symptoms, general health, socioeconomic factors, and general dietary habits was used. Two (prospective, i.e., looking to the future) four-day dietary records were used to estimate average daily nutrient intake.[185] A total of 181 healthy Danish women volunteers, aged 20-45 years, not pregnant and not using oral contraceptives, were selected. The results of the survey analysis indicated that dietary habits were correlated with menstrual pain. *Women with the highest intake of omega-3 fatty acids had the mildest symptoms during menstruation.* The researchers consider the results to be highly significant in support of the hypothesis that a higher intake of marine omega-3 fatty acids correlates with milder menstrual symptoms.

OSTEOPOROSIS

Who would suspect that fatty acid nutrition would have an effect on bone health? Believe it or not, that's what research is indicating. Lab animals lacking the essential fatty acids develop severe osteoporosis, plus kidney and arterial calcification. This disease process is similar to what is seen in osteoporosis among the elderly. In senior citizens, the loss of bone calcium is linked to calcium deposits in other tissues, especially arteries and kidneys. Even more disturbing, recent mortality studies find calcium deposition in these soft tissues much more dangerous than osteoporosis itself. Why is that? Surprisingly, the majority of deaths in women with osteoporosis are due to vascular disease, not fractures or other bone problems.

Essential fatty acids increase calcium absorption from the intestines. This is accomplished by enhancing the effects of vitamin D, which reduces calcium loss in urine, increases calcium deposition into bone, improves bone strength, and optimizes the manufacture of collagen, the bones' connective tissue. All of these actions help to reduce the deposition of calcium in undesirable places. Fatty acid effects on calcium metabolism may offer new approaches to osteoporosis and associated vascular and kidney disease.

A South African team recently studied the effect of fatty acids on calcium metabolism in the elderly.[186] 65 women whose average age was 79.5, with a foundation diet low in calcium, were randomly assigned to gamma-linolenic acid (GLA, an omega-6 fatty acid) plus EPA or a coconut oil placebo. They also received 600 mg of calcium carbonate daily. Biomarkers of bone formation and degradation, as well as bone mineral density (BMD), were measured at the beginning of the study and at six, 12, and 18 months. 21 patients continued with the treatment for a second 18-month period. At eighteen months, biomarkers indicated a decrease in bone turnover and the beneficial effects of calcium given to all the patients.

However, lower spine and thigh bone BMDs showed different effects in the two groups. During the first 18 months, spinal density remained the same in the treatment group, but declined 3.2 percent in the placebo group. Thigh bone density actually increased 1.3 percent in the treatment group, but decreased 2.1 percent in the placebo group. During the second 18 months, with all patients on active treatment, lumbar spine density increased 3.1 percent in patients who remained on active treatment, and 2.3 percent in patients who switched to active treatment. Thigh BMD in the group that switched showed an increase of 4.7 percent. Investigators concluded that GLA and EPA have beneficial effects on bone and that they are safe for prolonged use.

MENOPAUSE—ESSENTIAL FATS
OFTEN LACKING IN WOMEN'S DIETS

Premenopause is marked by hormonal fluctuations associated with early menopause-related changes; women usually maintain regular menstrual cycles. *Perimenopause* is the transition between the premenopausal phase and menopause and is characterized by changes in estrogen levels, irregular menstrual cycles, and increased menopausal symptoms.

Many women experiencing early signs of menopause or who have PMS symptoms will benefit tremendously from specific omega-3 therapy. Essential fatty acids are required for the production of hormones, calcium absorption, and the absorption of fat-soluble vitamins that nourish our skin, nerves and mucous membranes. These same fats further benefit women's immune, cardiovascular, reproductive and central nervous system health. In addition, they are both transformational and beautifying for women's skin, hair and nails.

Volumes of scientific studies on the omega-3 fatty acids have shown how important these are for women's overall health. Not only have omega-3s been shown to relieve depression, fatigue, and allergies, they are a specific healing agent for skin conditions like eczema, psoriasis, acne, and dry skin.

There is also emerging research that suggests omega-3s are vital for the prevention of breast cancer, a disease that currently strikes one in eight women (see Part II, Chapter 2: Reduce Cancer Risk with Omega-3 Fatty Acids).

PAINFUL MENSTRUATION

Dysmenorrhea, or painful menstruation, is classified as either primary or secondary. Primary dysmenorrhea generally occurs within a couple of years of the first menstrual period. The pain tends to decrease with age and very often eases after childbirth. Secondary dysmenorrhea is commonly a result of endometriosis, starts later in life, and tends to increase in intensity over time.

As many as half of menstruating women are affected by dysmenorrhea, and of these, about ten percent have severe dysmenorrhea, which greatly limits activities for one to three days each month.[187]

In one double-blind trial, fish oil led to a statistically significant thirty-seven percent drop in menstrual symptoms.[188] In that report, adolescent girls with dysmenorrhea were given 1,080 mg of EPA and 720 mg of DHA per day for two months to achieve this result. Other trials have yet to study the relationship between fish oil and dysmenorrhea. To achieve the approximate level of EPA and DHA used in this trial often takes six grams fish oil per day.

BEAUTIFUL SKIN WITH OMEGA-3S

The human body desperately requires dietary fats—the proper fats—for ultimate skin beauty. But too many women have cut out *all* fats—and that's dangerous to their beauty quest.

Not surprisingly, up to seven percent of the population suffers from skin conditions such as eczema, which is characterized by chronically itchy, inflamed skin that is dry, red, and scaly. Another two to four percent of people suffer from psoriasis, which is characterized by sharply bordered reddened plaques covered with overlapping silvery scales.[189]

Yet, although the skin requires fats and oils, what it doesn't need is excess amounts of saturated fats, partially hydrogenated vegetable oils or other types of highly processed fats used to flavor and texturize convenient fast foods.

Beautiful skin requires the *proper* fats in order to maintain optimal skin cell membrane fatty acids and the proper balance of local tissue hormones called prostaglandins. The beauty-enhancing oils (essential fatty acids) from omega-3 fatty acids are absolutely critical to the vitality and youthfulness of your skin.

SKIN REQUIRES CONSTANT SUPPLY
OF ESSENTIAL FATTY ACIDS

Prostaglandins, which strongly influence skin health, are the body's local chemical messengers that govern many processes, including inflammation. They are not stored in the body but must be constantly synthesized from essential fatty acids that are taken in from the diet and deposited in cell membranes.

The consequences of an EFA deficiency can be devastating to the skin. When the body lacks EFAs, this deficit leads to an imbalance in prostaglandins, resulting in skin problems such as dryness, itching, eczema, scaling, and thinning. Beyond skin, nails may crack, and hair will become discolored and thin.

Psoriasis may be one of the skin's indicators of systemic inflammation. Research from the Department of Dermatology at the University of California, Davis shows that omega-3s may be particularly beneficial in cases of psoriasis. Arachidonic acid, an omega-6 fatty acid found in cell membranes from omega-6 dietary sources, is turned into another pro-inflammatory chemical, leukotriene B4, which is known to accumulate in the lesions of psoriasis sufferers. Both EPA and gamma-linolenic acid (from evening primrose or borage oils) are both potent inhibitors of leukotriene B4 generation. "It seems reasonable, therefore, that adequate dietary supplementation with eicosapentaenoic acid or gamma-linolenic acid may offer a novel and nontoxic approach to suppressing cutaneous inflammatory disorders," notes UC Davis researcher V.A. Ziboh.[190]

Meanwhile, omega-3s are converted to less inflammatory prostaglandins and leukotrienes. Omega-3 fatty acids also inhibit the body's production of inflammation-causing arachidonic acid, the raw material for these pro-inflammatory compounds. Arachidonic acid is usually found in animal foods together with saturated fat. Omega-3s favorably inhibit the body's conversion of arachidonic acid to pro-inflammatory prostaglandins.

Let's look at a few specific conditions.

Eczema

Eczema is a common skin condition characterized by an itchy, red rash. Many skin diseases cause somewhat similar rashes, so it is important to have the disease properly diagnosed before it can be treated.

Eczema can be triggered by allergies. Most children with eczema have food allergies, according to data from double-blind research. A doctor should be consulted to determine if allergies are a factor. Once the trigger for the allergy has been identified, avoidance of the allergen can lead to significant improvement.

It has been reported that when heavy coffee drinkers with eczema avoided coffee, eczema symptoms improved.[191] In this study, the reaction was to coffee—not caffeine, indicating an allergic reaction to the former. People with eczema who are using a hypoallergenic diet to investigate food allergies should avoid coffee as part of this trial.

Ten grams of fish oil providing 1.8 g of EPA per day were given to a group of eczema sufferers in a double-blind trial. After 12 weeks, those using the fish oil experienced significant improvement.[192,193] According to the researchers, fish oil may be effective because it reduces levels of leukotriene B4, a substance that has been linked to eczema.[194] The eczema-relieving effects of fish oil may require taking ten pills per day for at least 12 weeks; smaller amounts of fish oil have been shown to lack efficacy.[195] One trial reported that fish oil was barely more effective than the vegetable placebo (a 30 percent versus 24 percent improvement, respectively).[196] As vegetable oil has previously been reported to have therapeutic activity, the apparent negative outcome of this trial should not dissuade people with eczema from considering fish oil.

Psoriasis

Psoriasis is a common disease that produces silvery, scaly plaques on the skin. A dermatologist should be consulted to confirm the diagnosis of psoriasis.

To begin, some dietary changes may be helpful. Ingestion of alcohol appears to be a risk factor for psoriasis in men, but not women.[197,198] It would therefore be prudent for men with psoriasis to drink moderately, if at all. Anecdotal evidence suggests that people with psoriasis may improve on a hypoallergenic diet.[199]

In a double-blind study, fish oil (ten grams per day) was found to improve the skin lesions of psoriasis.[200] In another study, supplementing with 3.6 g per day of purified EPA reduced the severity of psoriasis after two to three months.[201,202] That amount of EPA is contained in about 20 g of fish oil.

Additional research is needed to determine whether fish oil itself, or some of its components, are more effective for individuals with psoriasis. One study showed that applying a preparation containing ten percent fish oil directly to psoriatic lesions twice daily resulted in improvement after seven weeks. In addition, promising results were reported from a double-blind study in which people with chronic plaque-type psoriasis received 4.2 g of EPA and 4.2 g of DHA or placebo intravenously each day for two weeks. Thirty-seven percent of those receiving the essential fatty acid infusions experienced greater than fifty percent reduction in the severity of their symptoms.[204]

Supplementing with fish oil also may help prevent the increase in blood levels of triglycerides that occurs as a side effect of certain drugs used to treat psoriasis (e.g., etretinate and acitretin).[205]

CHAPTER 8

Arthritis–A Remedy with Omega-3 Oils

Arthritis is an inflammation of the joints and surrounding tendons and liga-ments. Among the oldest known afflictions of human beings, it can affect vir-tually any joint. According to the National Institutes of Health (NIH), arthritis' detrimental effects range from slight pain, stiffness and swelling of the joints to crippling and disability. There are two primary types of arthritis: osteoarthritis and rheumatoid arthritis.

Osteoarthritis is caused by the degeneration of the cartilage tissue in the large, weight bearing joints of the body—mainly the hips and knees.

Rheumatoid arthritis is thought to be caused by an autoimmune condition in which the body's immune system attacks its own joint tissues. With this condition, joints—most commonly the small joints of the hand—become tender, swollen, and, after years of damage, even deformed. It is not uncommon for an arthritis sufferer to have varying degrees of both types of arthritis. Regardless of the type, the end result is pain and inflammation at the sight of affliction.

This fact has led to the popularity of over-the-counter and prescription medica-tions to combat inflammation, and thus diminish pain. Such medicines as aspirin and nonsteroidal anti-inflammatory drugs (NSAIDs) come with long-term side effects, including a worsening of the arthritic condition; they work by interfering with the enzymes that produce the hormone-like compounds called prostaglandins. We can suggest another avenue of healing which may be much more safe, involving the use of omega-3 fatty acids to regulate the body's inflammatory processes. Omega-3 oils have been scientifically proven to be powerful anti-inflammatory agents.

REMOVE OBSTACLES TO HEALING

The clinical experience of many naturopathic physicians and holistic medical doc-tors indicates that it is imperative to rule out food allergies and sensitivities that can exacerbate the symptoms of arthritis. This is especially problematic in persons suffering from what is called the "leaky gut" phenomenon, in which significant amounts of undigested proteins enter the bloodstream, triggering inflammatory immune responses. As with ADHD, the elimination diet, removing especially the most commonly consumed foods such as wheat, dairy and cheese, can give amazing relief in some patients. An experienced health professional familiar with its application should be consulted.[206]

OMEGA-3 FATTY ACIDS— POWERFUL ANTI-INFLAMMATORY AGENTS

A family of local tissue hormones called prostaglandins and leukotrienes regulates the body's local inflammatory response. If too much of the omega-6 fatty acid called arachidonic acid is located on cell membranes, the enzymes that synthesize prostaglandins and leukotrienes will convert arachidonic acid into pro-inflammatory

FYI: Ingesting All the Wrong Kinds of Fats

Most people today ingest high amounts of omega-6 rich oils, such as corn, safflower, and sunflower, as well as grain-fed animal meats, which lead to the production of inflammatory prostaglandins, worsening the symptoms of arthritis and other inflammatory conditions.

compounds. On the other hand, if there is a preponderance of EPA within cell membranes, the enzymes will convert arachidonic acid to non-inflammatory prostaglandins and leukotrienes. Thus, the non-inflammatory prostaglandins and leukotrienes are produced from omega-3 fatty acid dietary sources. The high content of omega-3 fatty acids in these sources stimulates the body's production of non-inflammatory prostaglandins.

THE CASE FOR OMEGA-3 OILS

As we mentioned, our nemesis arachidonic acid is the fatty acid that accumulates on cell membranes when people consume a diet high in common omega-6 fatty acids from vegetable oils and grain (corn)-fed livestock. Tissue enzymes convert arachidonic acid into pro-inflammatory local hormones called prostaglandins and leukotrienes. Both EPA and DHA, the fatty acids of fish oils, are converted into non-inflammatory prostaglandins and leukotrienes. Researchers at the Albany Medical College and the State University of New York conducted a small, non-randomized, double-blinded, placebo-controlled, crossover trial using fish oil in addition to conventional pharmaceuticals. Fish oils proved to be quite superior to the placebo in relieving the symptoms of rheumatoid arthritis, as well as reducing the production of pro-inflammatory leukotrienes. The dosage involved a daily total of 2.7 g EPA and 1.8 g DHA during treatment periods of 14 weeks. The researchers concluded that fish oil relieves arthritis symptoms, but at least twelve weeks of intervention are required before the benefits are apparent.[207]

REDUCTION OF DIETARY OMEGA-6
FATS IS CRITICAL TO SUCCESS

This beneficial effect of dietary omega-3 fatty acids and supplements is significantly reduced when the diet is high in omega-6 linoleic acid. An Australian research team conducted a controlled experiment involving 30 male volunteers given 1.6 g EPA and 0.32 g DHA daily. Half the volunteers ate a diet high in linoleic acid by using margarine and polyunsaturated vegetable oils for cooking. The other half used butter and olive oil, which are low in linoleic acid. After four weeks, the incorporation of EPA into white blood cells was superior with a diet low in omega-6 fatty acids. Omega-6 laden margarine and polyunsaturated vegetable oils had inhibited the incorporation of omega-3s into tissue membranes. Therefore, omega-6s need to be reduced in the diet in order to obtain maximum benefit from fish oil omega-3s.[208]

REDUCING THE NEED FOR
PHARMACEUTICAL DRUGS

Belgian researchers studied the effect of long-term fish oil supplementation in rheumatoid arthritis patients. Sixty patients completed the 12-month, double-blind, randomized study that divided patients into three groups receiving daily supplements with either 2.6 g of omega-3s, or 1.3 g of omega-3s plus 3 g of olive oil, or 6 g of olive oil (placebo). All patients continued their pharmaceutical arthritis medicines. 53 percent of patients in the fish oil group showed significant overall improvement, compared to 10 percent in the placebo group and 33 in the fish plus olive oils group. 47 percent of the fish oil group were also able to reduce pharmaceutical dosing, compared to 15 percent on the placebo and 29 percent using both oils. The Belgian researchers concluded that long-term intake of fish oil benefits rheumatoid arthritis (RA) patients significantly and may reduce their need for drug medicines.[209]

An American team decided to really put fish oil to the test. Researchers at the

Albany Medical College enrolled 66 patients with active RA into a double-blind, placebo-controlled study. The purpose of the investigation was to determine:

- whether fish oil supplements will allow the discontinuation of non-steroidal anti-inflammatory drugs (NSAIDs) in RA patients;
- clinical efficacy of high-dose omega 3 fatty acid fish oil supplements in RA patients;
- and the effect of fish oil supplements on the production of multiple cellular chemical messengers linked to inflammation.

While taking diclofenac (75 mg twice daily), patients took either 130 mg/kg/day of omega-3 fatty acids or nine capsules/day of corn oil. Placebo diclofenac was substituted at week 18 or 22, and fish oil supplements were continued for eight weeks (to week 26 or 30). In the fish oil group, there were significant decreases in the number of tender joints, duration of morning stiffness, physician's and patient's assessment of overall arthritis activity, and physician's evaluation of pain. In the corn oil group, there was no clinical improvement. The decrease in the number of tender joints remained significant eight weeks after the fish oil patients discontinued the drug and was significant compared with patients receiving corn oil. Chemical messengers of inflammation also declined in the fish oil group. The investigators concluded that fish oil improves the symptoms of RA and that some patients who take fish oil are able to discontinue NSAIDs without experiencing a symptomatic flare-up.[210]

DATA POOLING

Despite these studies that have demonstrated how well fish oil alleviates rheumatoid arthritis, their small size minimizes their impact on conventional treatment of arthritis. Metanalysis and meganalysis are techniques that pool the results of small well-designed studies in order to see what conclusions can be drawn from the preponderance of evidence. A Harvard Medical School research group conducted a metanalysis of small clinical studies of the efficacy of fish oil in rheumatoid arthritis. The metanalysis included 10 double blind, randomized, placebo-controlled studies. The studies involved a total of 368 patients who took fish oil supplements for at least three months. The analyses demonstrated that fish oil supplementation for three months significantly reduced tender joint count and morning stiffness, compared to dietary control oils. No statistically significant changes were observed for the other measured indicators of disease severity.[211]

THE ROLE OF ANTIOXIDANTS

Inflammatory processes generate free radicals, which perpetuate inflammation. Consequently, the application of free radical scavengers—antioxidants—is well indicated in RA. Dietary antioxidants include vitamin C (ascorbate) and vitamin E (tocopherols). Beneficial effects of high doses have been reported, especially in osteoarthritis. Carotenes and selenium might also be helpful.[212]

GETTING OPTIMAL RESULTS WITH FISH OILS

How can arthritis patients use fish oil fatty acids to get the greatest symptomatic relief? Dr. Joel Kremer of the Albany Medical College recently published a summary of the current understanding concerning fish oil fatty acids and rheumatoid arthritis. Based on his review of the literature, Dr. Kremer concludes that dosing at three to six grams

Did You Know?
Modern Dietary Foibles

The high prevalence of arthritis and other inflammatory conditions may be due largely to the fact that we ingest far too much omega-6 rich oils and animal meats in proportion to the amount of omega-3 fatty acids we consume. This shift in dietary ingestion of omega-3 to omega-6 has been well documented over the past 100 years. One study concluded that arthritics suffer from a 40 percent deficiency in essential fatty acids compared to arthritis-free Americans, and a far higher deficiency compared to people from non-industrialized nations.

daily of EPA / DHA for at least 12 weeks or more is necessary to derive the expected benefits.[213] In addition, as the authors of this book have seen and the literature has confirmed, the benefits will be enhanced if omega-6 dietary sources are reduced.

NATURAL ALTERNATIVE TO
ANTI-INFLAMMATORY MEDICATIONS

Unlike medications that interfere with prostaglandin metabolism, omega-3 oils naturally temper the inflammatory prostaglandins, resulting in a decrease in painful inflammation. The difference between the drug approach and that taken with omega-3 oils is that the oils do not come with the common side effects linked to the medications. Not only do the omega-3 oils come without side effects, but they also have been medically proven to benefit as many as 50 other common afflictions. In other words, don't be surprised if you notice other health improvements beyond your expectations. Beyond the power of regulating prostaglandins, omega-3 oils have been found to modulate the immune system, lessening the severity of autoimmune conditions, including rheumatoid arthritis.

THE DOCTORS' PRESCRIPTION

There have been many studies to validate the use of essential fatty acids such as the omega-3s in arthritic conditions.[214,215,216]

The difference between flax and fish oils is the type of omega-3s they provide. Flax provides omega-3 in the form of alpha-linolenic acid. Wild ocean fish oil supplies omega-3 fatty acids in the form of EPA and DHA. The types of omega-3 fatty acids in fish oils have a much better record of documentation for enhancing the body's healing response in cases of arthritis. Due to dietary deficiencies in nutrients that assist the enzymes that convert ALA to EPA, as well as trans fatty acids that deactivate those enzymes, the long-term diets of many arthritics have encumbered this conversion. For this reason, we would definitely suggest that consumers use high-quality, lab-tested fish oil capsules.

While the causes of arthritis are truly multifactorial, part of the problem can clearly be identified as a lack of omega-3. Foods such as wild fish and fish oil has been found to increase tissue levels of the valuable omega-3s, as well as favorably augment non-inflammatory prostaglandins, averting inflammatory conditions. A practical dietary approach would be to lessen the intake of potentially inflammatory omega-6 oils, as well as grain-fed animal products, and supplement your diet with anti-inflammatory omega-3 oils. An average daily dose of fish oil is one-to-two tablespoons a day and will prove to be an important dietary consideration for those suffering from arthritic inflammatory conditions.

CHAPTER 9

Omega-3s & Asthma

Between 20 and 25 percent of all children suffer from one or more symptoms of asthma. Asthma may respond to dietary modification, reducing the need for pharmaceutical drugs. High dietary intake of linoleic acid (omega-6) may exacerbate asthma symptoms.

INCREASES IN PREVALENCE AND DEATHS

Asthma is the leading chronic illness of childhood, is responsible for substantial infant morbidity, and has a significant impact on the use of health resources, say researchers from the Department of Pediatrics at the University of Washington and the Center for Health Studies at Group Health Cooperative in Seattle.[217]

Other researchers note that asthma prevalence in children has increased 58 percent since 1980 and that mortality has increased by 78 percent.[218] Interestingly, the burden of the disease is most acute in urban areas and among racial and ethnic minority populations; hospitalization and morbidity rates for non-whites are more than twice those for whites.

Although studies illustrating the causal effects between outdoor air pollution and asthma prevalence are scant, air pollution appears to significantly worsen symptoms among children already with the disease. Decreased lung function, bronchial inflammation and other asthma symptoms such as recurrent wheezing, breathlessness, chest tightness and coughing have been associated with exposure to particulates, ozone, smoke, sulfur dioxide, and nitric oxide.

Fish oil may be an excellent natural medicine for helping children with asthma better cope with their condition. Supplementing an asthmatic child's diet with omega-3 oils is not only easy to do for parents; it is one of the most positive, cost-effective and beneficial natural approaches to asthma. In some cases, using omega-3 may help children to reduce or eliminate their need for asthma medication.

Omega-3 fatty acids help prevent asthma attacks by reducing the local tissue production of pro-inflammatory compounds that prime the tissue for hypersensitivity reactions to substances and conditions in the environment. The benefit of omega-3s in asthmatic patients will be enhanced, as usual, by a reduction in the intake of the common sources of omega-6s.

HOW OMEGA-3S HELP

Research in the past decade has revealed the importance of inflammation of the airways in asthma and successful clinical therapies aimed at reducing chronic inflammation. Asthma is associated with the local tissue production of pro-inflammatory fatty acid metabolites called leukotrienes, secreted by the immune system's white blood cells (leukocytes) as a reaction to common environmental allergens and pollutants, including house dust mites, animal dander, cockroach, fungal spores, pollens, and industrial airborne contaminants.

Ordinarily, white blood cells defend the body against infecting organisms and foreign agents, both in the tissues and in the bloodstream itself. But in persons with asthma, the white blood cells tend to produce excess amounts of inflammatory leukotrienes.

One way to counter the body's excess production of leukotrienes is to increase the intake of omega-3 fatty acids. The omega-3 fatty acids cause cells to produce more non-inflammatory leukotrienes and less of those that are prone to increase inflammatory processes. An expert in the *American Journal of Clinical Nutrition* notes that this shift from pro-inflammatory to non-inflammatory leukotrienes is directly related to relief from asthma symptoms.[219]

Some types of wild fish—such as mackerel and wild Pacific salmon—are a rich source of omega-3 fatty acids, and it has been shown that children who eat fish more than once a week have only one-third the risk of asthma compared with children who do not eat fish regularly.[220]

NOT A SUBSTITUTE FOR EMERGENCY MEDICINES

As preventive tools, omega-3s can never substitute for the life-saving emergency pharmaceuticals asthmatics sometimes need. These patients should always have them available for urgent situations. In addition, the use of dietary modifications to achieve a reduction in asthmatic tendency must be coordinated with the patient's health professional. Nevertheless, many patients have benefited from the use of these natural compounds in a way that reduces their dependency of drug therapy.

FIRST THINGS FIRST—
OPTIMAL HYDRATION

Histamine is a major mediator of asthma. It is released by mast cells located on the mucous membranes of the respiratory system. The biological function of histamine is to facilitate the movement of the immune system's white blood cells to sites of invasion by microbes. Animal studies indicate that increasing water consumption decreases histamine. As a result, asthma symptoms are reduced. Of course, identifying and eliminating allergens and triggering agents to which a person is sensitive is a major aspect of intervention. Nevertheless, in addition to vitamin B_{12}, omega-3 fatty acids, flavonoids, botanical medicines, homeopathics, and other natural healing modalities, pure water should be a key component of regimens for hypersensitivity states, such as asthma.[221]

THE PREVENTIVE POWER
OF WILD FISH

Researchers at the University of Sydney, Australia noted epidemiological studies suggesting that consumption of fish more than once a week reduces the risk of developing airway hypersensitivity. They decided to study the effect of fish consumption on asthmatic attacks. The investigation involved 574 children aged eight to eleven years. Parents completed detailed questionnaires about the frequency of eating for more than 200 foods over a one-year period. The children were evaluated for current asthma tendency. The researchers found that children who regularly ate fresh, fatty fish (e.g., mullet, orange roughy, Atlantic salmon or rainbow trout), containing more than two percent fat, had only one-quarter of the risk of developing asthma than did children who rarely or never ate oily fish. Risk reduction held firm even after adjusting for such risk factors as parental asthma history and smoking, early respiratory infections, ethnicity, and place of birth. Non-oily fish and canned fish were not protective. The researchers believe that EPA may prevent asthma development or reduce its severity by reducing airway inflammation and hyper-responsiveness.[222] Studies like these make us wonder how much healthier the children would be if mothers had consumed more fresh wild fish during pregnancy and nursing.

OMEGA-3 FATTY ACIDS
AS PREVENTIVE TOOLS

Researchers at the University of Wyoming have found that adjusting the dietary intake of polyunsaturated fatty acids may reduce asthma symptoms in many patients. Their clinical trial involved 26 non-smoking asthma sufferers aged 19 to 25 years. The usual intake of omega-6s was determined for each participant at the beginning of the study and after one month. For the first month, participants took fish oil capsules containing enough EPA and DHA to adjust their intake ratio of omega-3s to omega-6 to 0.1:1. During the second month the omega-3 to omega-6 ratio was elevated to 0.5:1. The average fish oil intake required to produce the 0.5:1 ratio was 3.3 g daily. More than 40 percent of patients experienced a significant improvement in breathing ability and decreased tendency to asthma attacks while supplementing with high levels of fish oil. The researchers conclude that omega-3 supplements may be an effective therapy for asthma.

What is particularly noteworthy about this study is the care with which dosing of omega-3 was individually adjusted to achieve a desired intake ratio. This kind of design is not done often enough to really help us refine our healing interventions with patients. The lack of this kind of sophistication in prescribing may explain why there have been some studies that have failed to demonstrate clinical efficacy for omega-3 fatty acids.[223]

In a third study, the effects of EPA were studied on asthma symptoms. In this Japanese study, patients were given EPA (1,800 milligrams per day) and they recorded signs and symptoms in an asthma diary during a two-week observation period. Administration of EPA was associated with improvements in symptoms of asthma and improved lung function. Thus, the researchers concluded that this omega-3 fatty acid "may be useful in patients with asthma."[224]

Recent studies have shown that omega-3 fatty acids have has a profound ability to inhibit the generation of pro-inflammatory leukotrienes by the white blood cells in asthmatics. Japanese researchers reporting in the *International Archives of Allergy and Immunology* compared the clinical features of asthmatics that had received oil supplements rich in omega-3s against a group not receiving the nutrient.[225] The scientists found that after only two weeks of supplementation, generation of pro-inflammatory leukotrienes by white blood cells known as leukocytes decreased significantly in the intervention group. In contrast, the production of pro-inflammatory leukotrienes "increased significantly" among persons not receiving the supplement. Even more intriguing, after only four weeks of dietary supplementation, lung function among the intervention group was significantly enhanced by the addition. Blood levels of total cholesterol, low-density lipoprotein (LDL) cholesterol and triglycerides were significantly decreased by dietary supplementation. The researchers concluded that dietary supplementation suppresses the generation of leukotrienes and can have many beneficial therapeutic effects among asthma patients.

The same scientific team conducted another study where the effects of omega-3s on bronchial asthma were compared with the effects of corn oil for lung function and generation of leukotrienes. (Corn oil, as mentioned previously in this book, is the most widely consumed vegetable oil that stimulates the production of pro-inflammatory fatty acids). In this study, 14 persons with asthma were divided randomly into two equal groups: one consumed omega-3s acid and the other corn oil for four weeks. Those receiving corn oil generated more pro-inflammatory leukotrienes, while those whose diets were supplemented by omega-3s decreased them. Again, lung function was better among persons receiving the alpha-linolenic acid. These results suggest that omega-3 supplementation "is useful for the treatment of asthma in terms of suppression of [pro-inflammatory leukotriene] generation by leucocytes, and improvement of pulmonary function."[226]

RESOLVING SCIENTIFIC CONFLICTS

Several studies using fish oil fatty acids EPA and DHA have not demonstrated any significant improvement in asthma symptoms.[227,228,229] As mentioned previously, any study design that employs olive oil as a placebo may be problematic because olive oil may not be as inert; therefore, it is an unsuitable placebo. In addition, insufficient time is allotted to allow the full potential of fish oil to manifest. At least three months—sometimes six or more months—are necessary before the full potency of fish oil intervention manifests.

One study even had the fish oil treatment group use margarine, even though it was made using omega-3 oils. Unfortunately, the manufacture of the artificial man-made fat we call *margarine* requires the heating of oil in the presence of a catalyst, such as nickel. Hydrogen gas is then bubbled through the catalyzed, heated oil so that enough of the unsaturated bonds are saturated with hydrogen to render the product solid at room temperature, like butter.

The problem with hydrogenated oils is that they are modified and damaged fatty acids. When you hydrogenate omega-3 oil, you no longer have omega-3 fatty acids. They have hydrogenated to less unsaturated forms, some of which are unmanageable by the body. In addition, the heat of the process causes some of the fatty acids to re-configure from their natural forms into a natural and harmful trans-fatty acids. And on top of all this, the processing of fatty acids in this manner can accelerate peroxidation, increasing the risk of generating damaging free radicals when the fatty are consumed. Why study designers don't avoid these pitfalls is puzzling and disappointing.

THE DOCTORS' PRESCRIPTION

- Asthma is often thought of as a debilitating childhood disease. It shouldn't be. There are tremendous opportunities to aid children with asthma.
- Be sure to drink lots of pure water to optimally hydrate respiratory membranes. This is particularly important in exercise-induced asthma.
- Supplementing the asthmatic child's diet with fish oil daily can help to provide the foundation for success. Consumption of wild fish rich in omega-3 fatty acids can also help.

FYI: Something to Think About:
Don't Let Asthma Leave You Breathless

About one of every five athletes who participated in the 1996 Summer Olympic Games in Atlanta had a personal history of asthma, had symptoms that suggested asthma, or took asthma medications, note researchers from the University of Iowa in Iowa City and the United States Olympic Committee in Colorado.[230] This should tell us that when proper steps are taken children with asthma can go on to achieve great things, even in elite sports competition.

CHAPTER 10

Oil Gets in Your Eyes

Age-related macular degeneration (AMD) is the leading cause of irreversible blindness in adults. The macula is the part of the retina of the eye that receives light images passing through the center of the lens. It is the highly sensitive part of the retina that allows us to see the precise detail of our central vision. Macular degeneration arises from either the accumulation of the cellular debris of aging (dry type) or the development of an undesirable network of new blood vessels, which may hemorrhage into the retina (wet type). The wet type is treated with laser surgery; the dry type can be prevented or treated by natural means.

Antioxidant nutrients, especially carotenoids such as lutein, zeaxanthin, and lycopene, as well as zinc and selenium, are helpful preventive nutritional interventions. Omega-3 fatty acids also have an equally important role to play. The reason becomes clear from previous discussions in this book when we consider that nervous tissue is the type of tissue that comprises the retina; therefore, one might suspect that our old friends EPA, and especially DHA, would be favorable to nerve cells of the retina. Let's see if the research supports this concept.

Researchers at Harvard Medical School evaluated the relationship between the intake of total and specific types of fat and the risk for advanced AMD.[231] Scientists designed a multi-center case-control study that included 349 persons (55 to 80 years of age) with advanced, neovascular stage AMD (these patients were diagnosed within one year of their enrollment). The controls included 504 individuals with other, non-AMD eye diseases. Higher vegetable fat intake, as well as that of monounsaturated and polyunsaturated fats, was linked to a greatly elevated risk for AMD.

Higher consumption of omega-6s (especially linoleic acid) was also associated with a higher risk for AMD. Conversely, a higher intake of omega-3 fatty acids was associated with a lower risk for AMD among persons eating diets low in linoleic acid, especially those high in fish. The Harvard researchers concluded that higher intake of specific types of fat—vegetable, monounsaturated and polyunsaturated fats and linoleic acid—rather than total fat intake may be associated with a greater risk for advanced AMD. Thus, we know that diets high in omega-3 fatty acids and fish are inversely associated with risk for AMD, especially when the intake of omega-6s (linoleic acid) is low.

An Australian team inquired whether the dietary intake of fat or fish is associated with age-related macular disease.[232] Their population study involved more than 3,000 people aged 49 years or older, out of which persons with AMD were identified. A self-administered food frequency questionnaire was used to ascertain intakes of dietary fat and fish. Researchers discovered a higher frequency of fish consumption was associated with decreased risk. Persons with higher intake of cholesterol were much more likely to have AMD. The investigators concluded that the amount and type of dietary fat intake might be linked to AMD.

NUTRITIONAL PRESCRIPTION

Overall, people with a healthy dietary balance of omega-3 and omega-6 fatty acids, and a higher intake of fish, are less likely to develop AMD; it would appear that EPA and DHA from fish, eaten four or more times weekly, may reduce the risk. Fish oil supplements are also suggested.

CHAPTER 11

Weight Loss with Omega-3 Oils

What about persons suffering from fat phobia? After all, omega-3 fatty acids are forms of fat, aren't they? Well, as people around the world are beginning to experience, the major contributing dietary factor in obesity is refined carbohydrates, not fat per se. For example, we know that in some parts of Italy, olive oil, a source of omega-9 fatty acids, constitutes forty percent of the caloric intake in some people without an increased risk of heart disease or obesity.

That does not mean that fat intake is not an issue, but it does mean that we need to be less phobic about fat in our diet and more informed about the kind of fat in our diet and how fat fits into an overall healthy lifestyle.

The body responds to each kind of fatty acid differently. Some fats contribute to obesity, cardiovascular disease, stroke and other degenerative diseases, while the omega-3s in flaxseed oil, fish oil, walnuts, and fatty wild fish can prevent and may even reverse these afflictions.

Instead of trying to fool the body with sugar-laden, no- or low-fat foods, wild fish and their oils, in the context of a responsible diet and exercise, work with the metabolic and physiologic processes of the body, resulting in natural weight loss and

Did You Know?
How Omega-3 Oils Aid Weight Loss
- Decrease cravings for fatty foods and sweets.
- Improve metabolism.
- Create satiety (feeling of fullness and satisfaction following a meal).
- Regulate blood sugar.
- Regulate insulin levels.
- Increase oxygen utilization.

maintenance. The omega-3 fatty acids have been identified as essential nutrients. This is to say that the body cannot convert other food sources into these compounds. As a result, your body actually craves and looks for these essential nutrients in the foods you eat. If they are not there, the body engages in compensatory mechanisms to survive under the stress of nutritional inadequacy.

FISH FOR WEIGHT LOSS

Obesity in patients with high blood pressure is associated with disturbances in blood lipids and insulin resistance, both of which are improved by weight management. Keeping this in mind, an Australian research team conducted a 16-week study on 69 obese, hypertensive patients to determine whether dietary fish enhances the effects of weight loss on serum lipids, glucose, and insulin.[233] While being treated for hypertension, patients were randomly assigned to a daily fish meal, a weight-loss regimen, the two regimens combined, or a control group. The patients' weight decreased by an average of 12.32 pounds. The fish plus weight-loss group showed the greatest improvement in lipids: triglycerides decreased by 38 percent and HDL cholesterol increased by 24 percent compared to the control group. The investigators concluded that incorporating a daily fish meal into a weight-loss regimen is more effective at improving both glucose-insulin metabolism and blood fat disturbances than either measure alone. They stated, "Cardiovascular risk is likely to be substantially reduced in overweight hypertensive patients with a weight-loss program incorporating fish meals rich in [omega]-3 fatty acids." Thus, overweight people who follow a weight loss program with exercise, can achieve better control over blood sugar and cholesterol by also eating fatty fish, or at least supplementing with fish oil capsules, that are rich in omega-3 fatty acids.

Did You Know?
Athletes Report These Benefits with Omega-3s

- Enhanced athletic performance.
- Improved stamina and endurance.
- Shortened recorded time from athletic events and strenuous workouts.
- Reliable source of energy without increasing body fat.
- Reduced muscle soreness after strenuous workouts.
- Increased uptake and utilization of oxygen.

The ideal method of taking omega-3 oils for purposes of weight loss or maintenance is in divided doses taken with each meal.

CHAPTER 12

Flaxseed Oil–The Vegetarian Omega-3 Choice

The many health benefits of a vegetarian diet have been well documented, including reduced risk of cardiovascular disease, some types of cancer, osteoporosis, diabetes, and many other conditions. But can a vegetarian diet be improved upon? We say yes. In fact, a surprising, newly uncovered nutritional deficiency could be plaguing vegetarians across the country.

Past and present research suggests that vegetarians may be deficient in a critical and essential nutrient identified as omega-3 fatty acids. Lower proportions of omega-3 fatty acids are found in the blood of vegetarians compared to omnivores (meat and vegetable eaters), note researchers from the Department of Food Science at RMIT University in Melbourne, Australia.

In a study by scientists from the Research Institute of Nutrition in Bratislava, Slovakia, the plasma profile of fatty acids was examined in a group of children consisting of seven vegans (those who avoid anything derived from animals), fifteen lacto-ovo-vegetarians (those who consume dairy and eggs but no meat) and ten semi-vegetarians (those who avoid meats other than fish or chicken).[234] The children were 11 to 15 years old, and the average period of alternative nutrition was 3.4 years. The results were compared with a group of 19 omnivores. Values of omega-3 fatty acids in lacto-ovo-vegetarians were identical to those of omnivores whereas they were significantly increased in semi-vegetarians consuming fish twice a week. Due to the total exclusion of animal fats from the diet, vegans had significantly reduced values of omega-3 fatty acids.

The problem seems to be that the major sources of omega-3 fatty acids in the American diet are wild cold-water fish such as salmon, tuna, sardines, mackerel, as well as flaxseed. Obviously, wild ocean fish is not an option among vegetarians. Many vegetarians also consume foods very high in omega-3 fatty acid antagonists, such as sunflower and safflower oils, and very little flaxseed. So beneficial are such diets that even with this deficiency, they are excellent for human health among those agreeable to vegetarianism. The lesson here, however, is that while vegetarian diets are great, health-conscious individuals (and what vegetarian isn't aware of his or her own health?) can make their diet even better by addressing potential omega-3 fatty acid deficiencies.

A diet dominant in omega-6 fatty acids, and all but devoid of omega-3 fatty acids, causes a disproportionate amount of omega-6 fatty acids to accumulate in both animal and human tissues. Recent research all but blames this gross disproportion to the genesis of modern degenerative diseases including arthritis, cancer, heart attack, and stroke. Despite the trace amounts of omega-3 fatty acids present in vegetable foods, vegetarians have also been found to consume more omega-6 fatty acids in proportion to omega-3 than omnivores. This is probably due to the fact that vegetarians consume more omega-6 fatty acid-dominant grains as a staple to their diet than do omnivores.

Omnivores are also subject to omega-3 fatty acid-deficient diets, but to a slightly lesser extent. Ironically, when livestock are allowed to range-free and forage for their food, they ingest vegetable matter containing omega-3 fatty acids. Over time, the omega-3 fatty acids become concentrated in the animals' tissues. When products made from the flesh of these animals is consumed, omnivores unwittingly derive the benefit of the concentrated omega-3 fatty acids in the animal meat. This seeming advantage is becoming less of a factor as animals are kept penned up and fed grains that are primarily of the omega-6 variety, in order to grow the livestock to fulfill the market's timely demands. Omega-6 fatty acids are supplied in the diet at a percentage of 95 percent, meaning that the remaining five percent of our fat intake is omega-3 fatty acids, a woeful imbalance.

HEALTH IMPLICATIONS

In spite of the many benefits to be derived from a vegetarian diet, individual vegetarians may be at higher risk for ailments caused by a diet lacking omega-3s. These include:

- Aching, painful joints and muscles.
- Anovulatory menstrual cycles.
- Chest pains.
- Cracked nails.
- Depression.
- Dry hair and skin.
- Dry mucous membranes in the mouth, vagina, and other organs.
- Eczema, psoriasis and other skin conditions.
- Fatigue, malaise, lackluster energy, lack of endurance.
- Forgetfulness.
- Frequent colds and influenza.
- Inability to concentrate.
- Indigestion, gas, and bloating
- Irregular heartbeat.
- Lack of motivation.
- Premature wrinkling of skin.

As an example, a recent report in the *American Journal of Clinical Nutrition* found that male vegetarians actually had higher platelet aggregability than male omnivores. In other words, vegetarians were more likely to form blood clots that could trigger heart attacks or strokes.[235] Obviously, since vegetarians generally have a lower risk for heart disease or stroke, other facets of the vegetarian diet may minimize this particular negative aspect of circulatory.

THE DOCTORS' PRESCRIPTION

A vegetarian diet has been scientifically proven to prevent and possibly reverse some diseases of modern man. However, due to radical changes in food processing, manufacturing and dietary shifts, vegetarians have been found to be more deficient in essential omega-3 fatty acids than their omnivorous neighbors. This may predis-

FYI: Pregnant and Nursing Vegetarian Women Need to Up Their Omega-3 Fatty Acid Intake

This information is critical to women of childbearing age and those who are pregnant.[236] Lower levels of omega-3 fatty acids are also found in the milk of vegetarian mothers as well as in the red blood cells of their infants, compared to infants of omnivorous mothers or those bottle-fed on cow's milk formula. As a consequence, infants born to vegetarian mothers are likely to have lower stores of omega-3 fatty acids. Due to the importance of omega-3 fatty acids in the development of both the nervous system and visual acuity in infants, subtle effects on visual function may occur.

Omega-3 fatty acids are required for the normal development of the retina and central nervous system, notes Dr. Thomas Sanders, of the Nutrition, Food and Health Research Center, King's College in London. The developing fetus obtains omega-3 fatty acids via selective uptake from the mother's plasma. However, there are greater proportions of omega-6 fatty acids and lower proportions of omega-3 fatty acids in vegetarians compared with omnivores.

Lower concentrations of the omega-3 fatty acid docosahexaenoic acid (DHA) have been observed in the blood and artery phospholipids of infants of vegetarians. We know from primate studies that animals with an altered or impaired visual function tend to have a high ratio of omega-6 fatty acids to alpha-linolenic acid (the major omega-3 fatty acid in flaxseed oil).

Thus, it is smart to recommend to vegetarian women who are pregnant or nursing diets with a higher intake of omega-3 fatty acids and curbing excessive intakes of omega-6 fatty acids, says Dr. Sanders.

pose vegetarians to a variety of health ailments.

The optimal vegetarian diet should include a high quality source of omega-3 fatty acids, such as fresh flaxseed oil, to avoid omega-3 fatty acid deficiency and to provide a favorable balance of omega-6 to omega-3 fatty acids in the diet.

An all-natural vegetable source of omega-3 fatty acids may help to prevent and alleviate nutritional deficiency in vegetarians as well as omnivores. The most abundant source of vegetable omega-3 fatty acids comes from flaxseed oil. While it is possible to derive omega-3 in the diet from fish or flax, there is a foundational difference between the types of omega-3 fatty acids supplied by each source. While both sources are excellent, the good news for vegetarians is that the omega-3 fatty acid derived from vegetable sources such as flaxseed oil is a dietary essential. That is, once vegetable omega-3 fatty acid—alpha-linolenic acid—is ingested, the types of omega-3 fatty acids usually found in wild fish can be formed in the body (as long as trans-fatty acids are avoided and the vitamin-mineral co-factors for the converting enzymes are sufficient in the diet). In other words, it is not necessary, in most cases, for vegetarians to resort to consuming animal products to obtain the health benefits of nutritionally required omega-3 fatty acids. However, vegetarians should lower their intake of omega-6 fatty acids to facilitate the conversion of ALA to DHA and EPA, the omega-3s found in some cold-water fish.

The challenge is getting enough essential omega-3 fatty acids required for optimal health. The absolute best choice is unrefined, fresh, organic flaxseed oil. Flaxseed oil contains more omega-3 fatty acids than any other common commercial source.

Citing the potential for lower blood lipid levels of omega-3 fatty acids in vegetarians, the American Dietetic Association has advised "that vegetarians include a good source of ALA in their diet." The ADA goes on to list flaxseed oil as the richest source of ALA. The high amount of omega-3 fatty acids in flaxseed oil will help to balance out the excessive omega-6 fatty acids prevalent in the American diet. The recommended dosage of flaxseed is from one to two tablespoons a day. However, to receive the most benefit, consumers should make a conscious choice to remove extraneous sources of omega-6 fatty acids from the diet, such as refined foods, common vegetable oils (other than olive), and salad dressings high in omega-6 fatty acids. It would be prudent for vegetarians to use flaxseed oil, which has a very high percentage of omega-3 fatty acids as the basis for salad dressings, instead of sunflower, corn, safflower, and soy.

Some vegetarians might want to modify their dietary habits slightly to also include fish oil capsules.

CHAPTER 13

Caveat Emptor: Savvy Shopping Tips for Omega-3 Oils

Some experts say that the challenge of making a pure, high-quality fish oil product is much greater than making a good flaxseed oil product. With flax, if you start with organic flaxseed, as do our recommended products, one simply has to find an efficient, optimal way to squeeze the oil out of organic flaxseed. With fish, getting the oil out of the fish is just the beginning.

Fatty fish should be an ideal source of omega-3 fatty acids. However, most fish today are contaminated with environmental poisons, and farm-raised fish often lack adequate omega-3s due to their farm-fed diets that deprive them of some of the natural foods that would lead them to produce these valuable fatty acids. Another problem is that fatty fish become rancid immediately after death. (That is why Chinese people bring home their fish from the shop in a living state.) A third problem is that the fatty acids can be destroyed during the preparation of the fish, e.g. grilling or frying. These are some reasons why fish oils have been developed as a substitution for fish. As we will read on, however, all fish oils are not created equal.

PURE AIN'T SIMPLE: FINDING UNTAINTED FISH OILS

We live on a planet on the verge of ecological disaster. The great French ocean explorer Jacques Cousteau warned of the impending peril many years ago, but most Americans have ignored the warning. Most Americans do not comprehend how environmental pollution affects their personal lives. This obliviousness reminds us of the ostrich with its head in the sand, too fearful or aloof to engage impending danger until it gets its butt kicked really hard. We are not prophets of gloom and doom; we are merely stating the conclusions from our own observations and from those who spend their lives monitoring what is happening to the natural environment.

Since most Americans will not take action until it is made abundantly clear to them how issues affected their lives and those of their loved ones directly, we will discuss how the issue of environmental pollution affects you and yours directly in the context of omega-3 fatty acid nutrition. The world's oceans have been treated by humanity as sewers and cesspools. The industrialized nations have been the worst offenders, and since the United States is the greatest industrial power, the United States has been most injurious to Nature and should be a leader in pollution prevention (as it is).

For example, fishermen in Louisiana have to travel at least 50 miles into the Gulf of Mexico, away from the mouth of the Mississippi River, to find any fish to catch. The river's pollutants have decimated all fish habitat for a radius of 50 miles. And this is just one small example. When we consider the waste dumped into the oceans by all nations and their sailing vessels over the centuries—especially since the Industrial Revolution—the staggering scope of the problem becomes more apparent.

How does this problem affect Jane and John Doe on Main Street in the heartland of America? We have already seen the news reports of medical doctors advising patients not to eat large ocean fish due to the heavy contamination with mercury, whose effect on patients has been documented by diagnostic lab analysis. And this is just one pollutant doctors are testing for.

Many experts in the field of cancer research are convinced that the dramatic rise in cancer rates over the last century has been facilitated by carcinogenic pollution. Fish living in polluted waters are going to be polluted, so it obviously follows that oil extracted from such fish will also be polluted. The kind of poisons found in fish sounds like a list of what humans dump into the planet's waterways—mercury, lead, dioxin, and polychlorinated biphenyls (PCBs) are just some of the most notorious of the known pollutants. A recent Irish study publicized by the BBC indicates that a large number of the fish oil products sold in Europe contain three to six times the dioxin levels allowed under new European Union guidelines.

How can you be sure that your fish oil product is pure? Ask your retailer to request a copy of the lab analysis for the batch of product you want to buy. Any manufacturer who cannot retrieve that record from company files and fax it to your retailer within a few business days either never had the testing done or is too disorganized to be trusted to make a reliable product of consistent quality batch after batch.

Not all omega-3 products are the same. Extensive research in preparing this book has yielded substantial evidence that Icelandic production standards, and the clean, unpolluted waters from which their fish originate, ensure that their fish oils are produced under pharmaceutical-grade conditions with the finest quality and freshness. Their pharmaceutical-grade formulations also provide the highest concentration of quality ingredients. For example, it requires 100 gallons of health store-grade omega-3 fish oils to concentrate and produce just one gallon of pharmaceutical-grade quality fish oil.

These are the important factors we've found are important in comparing omega-3 production standards:

- The same exacting standards used for the production of prescription medications are utilized for the formulation, production and bottling.
- Manufactured under the Good Manufacturing Practice (GMP) regulations developed and promoted by the U.S. Food and Drug Administration. These regulations require that manufacturers of products, such as nutritional supplements, take proactive steps to ensure that their products are safe, pure, and effective.
- Meets ISO 9002 international quality standards, which require the highest levels of manufacturing standardization to ensure consistent quality.

Smart Shopper Tip
FYI: Supermarket vs. Custom Canned Troll-Caught Albacore

Most canned albacore found in supermarkets today come from very large canneries using assembly-line techniques to process huge quantities of tuna at a time. What most people do not realize is that albacore tuna sold by the major brands generally comes from larger, leaner albacore that has been cooked twice – and because of this, many natural juices, flavors, and healthful Omega-3s are lost in the process.

Here's how it works in the major commercial canneries: the albacore are received, inspected for quality, and then cooked whole on big racks. The cooked fish then travel down an assembly line, where workers remove the skin and pull the meat off the bones. During this process many of the natural juices, oils, and omega-3s drain off the meat and never make it into the cans. The pre-cooked meat is then placed in cans with water, broth, or vegetable oils before being cooked for the second time.

Because younger, smaller, troll-caught albacore naturally have more fat to start with, some of the healthful Omega-3s will still survive the high-volume industrial canning processes and make it to supermarket shelves. However, it is easier for big companies to work with the larger, leaner albacore in the assembly line environment. Starting out with less fatty fish right at the beginning means that virtually no omega-3s are left in the end product.

Meanwhile, with all the positive news about the health benefits of Omega-3s, demand is rising for custom canned albacore that are cooked just once in their natural juices to retain all of their omega-3 essential fatty acids and flavor.

Over the years many professional fishermen have been frustrated over having their catch processed into a product that doesn't taste like what they cook up themselves after a hard day's work. Many are also upset by the lack of labels pointing out younger

Continued on page 131...

- The quality of the ingredients should meet the exacting requirements of European Pharmacopoeia Standards.
- Products should be molecularly distilled, a state-of-the-art technology for removing impurities.
- Certified non-detectable levels of PCBs, heavy metals, mercury, pesticides, dioxins and other toxins.
- Independently tested for potency & purity.
- Uses advanced manufacturing technology to remove any fishy taste, but retains the full potency of the formulas.

We've discovered that omega-3 products from Iceland conform to each and every one these standards.

...Continued from page 130

troll-caught albacore in markets that have been overrun and flooded by older, larger albacore that have drier meat.

Some of these fishermen have therefore started paying to have some of their catch custom-canned and labeled to their specifications by small independent canneries. Just as "micro-breweries" offer gourmet beer and ales, these "micro-canners" specialize in providing limited quantities of gourmet albacore. While they cannot begin to compete with the high-volume, low-cost commercial albacore that dominate supermarket shelves today, some of their top-quality custom-canned albacore is starting to reach farmers markets, mail order catalogs, specialty shops, and the Internet. Most fishermen typically charge anywhere from three to six dollars per can, which is much higher than the major commercial brands, yet still comparable to other top-quality meats such as boneless free-range chicken breasts, veal, selected organic beef cuts, and the like.

So, is such custom canned albacore from fishermen worth the higher price? Absolutely. It is unlikely that the big brand-name commercial canneries can ever adjust their high-volume processing techniques for retaining natural juices and omega 3s, so the only public access to top-quality albacore will probably remain in the hands of enterprising fishermen who take special pride in their catch. Our advice: try some custom canned albacore and decide for yourself!

Visit *www.albatuna.com/sources/canned.htm* for a list of custom-canned albacore varieties available to the public by mail order, online, and in various locations in California, Oregon, and Washington. Each of the varieties included on the list comes from fishermen and small businesses that actively contribute to the American Fishermen's Research Foundation, which is dedicated to aiding, encouraging, promoting and supporting Pacific albacore tuna science and education projects.

Best Sources of Omega-3 Fatty Acids in Seafood

Fish	Amount per 100 g of raw fillet
Rainbow trout	1.1
Cisco	1.1
Pacific mackerel	1.1
Atlantic herring	1.1
Pacific herring	1.2
Sardine	1.2
American eel	1.2
Atlantic halibut	1.3
Sablefish	1.3
Atlantic salmon	1.4
Lake trout	1.4
Anchovy	1.4
Coho salmon	1.5
Pink salmon	1.5
Bluefin tuna	1.5
Atlantic mackerel	1.9
King salmon	1.9
Dogfish	1.9
Albacore tuna	2.1
Sockeye salmon	2.7

Source: Nettleton, Joyce A., *Seafood Nutrition—Facts Issues and Marketing of Nutrition in Fish and Shellfish.* Huntington, NY; Osprey Books, 1985.

CHAPTER 14

Putting It All Together

In order for the wealth of information provided in this book to be useful to the reader and consumer, the health-promoting properties of omega-3 fatty acids must be put into the context of a healthy lifestyle plan that can be followed with relative ease. Let's look at an overview of how omega-3s fits into a well-designed wellness plan. The following are what years of experience have taught to be the important cornerstones of health and wellness:

- Beneficial genetic inheritance.
- Positive mental attitude, open to new possibilities.
- Loving relationships.
- Optimal intake of pure water.
- Nutrient-dense diet, disciplined to the needs of the body and satisfaction of the palate, thoroughly masticated (chewed).
- Judiciously selected nutritional supplements.
- Moderate or greater regular exercise.
- Restful, refreshing sleep
- Meaningful self-affirming work.
- Pleasurable hobbies.
- Mind-expanding reading.
- Community service.
- Pollution-free environment.
- Spiritual faith and practice.
- Balanced interaction among all of the above elements with clearly defined priorities and effective stress management skills.

Because omega-3 fatty acids serve as nutrient sources, let's put them into a solid nutritional program. (Be sure to coordinate these recommendations with your health care professional.)

1) Drink copious amounts of pure water. The human body is an entity comprised of water compartmentalized into cells bounded by fatty acids. We must be optimally hydrated for optimal wellness. Do not trust your thirst to tell you when your body needs water. It is unreliable for optimal hydration and declines with age. Drink daily at least the number of fluid ounces equal to half the number of pounds the body weighs. (A 200-pound person should drink twelve eight-ounce cups daily.) As cold temperatures disturb biological processes, drink this water at room temperature or warmer. Minimize intake of artificial beverages, such as soft drinks. (See our recommended waters.)

2) Control caloric intake. Caloric intake must be balanced with physical activity to avoid obesity. Overeating can shorten the lifespan. Dietary self-discipline is essential to longevity. The only factor that has consistently enabled researchers to increase the lifespan of laboratory animals of all studied species is restricting caloric intake. That doesn't mean we have to starve ourselves. It does mean that we have to listen to our body's reliable signals and feedback indicating that we have gone beyond the realm of eating to live into the quagmire of living to eat.

The transition is so much easier when we learn to substitute organic whole foods for highly processed devitalized foods from which natural fiber and other nutrients have been removed. An organic, whole foods diet can be both delicious and satisfying in a way that allows people to maintain healthy body weight without feeling deprived of the tantalizing pleasure of eating imaginatively prepared cuisine.

3) Control quality and quantity of fats consumed. Limit total fat to less than 30 percent, and your saturated fat to less than ten percent, of your caloric intake. Maintain cholesterol intake to under 300 mg per day. Emphasize omega-3 sources while reducing omega-6s. Control consumption of alcohol, sugar, refined and processed foods, and salt.

Be sure to incorporate small, wild ocean fish in your diet. With the exception of wild game that some people are able to hunt, wild fish is the last source of wild food left in the diets of most people. Smaller fish have less toxins than the larger ones. As a rule of thumb, the larger the fish, the higher it is on the food chain, and the more concentrated environmental pollutants are in its tissues.

4) Design a nutrient-dense diet, rich in vitamins, minerals, and antioxidants. Eat five or more servings of fresh (organic is preferred) vegetables and fruits. Prefer vegetables and fruits with brilliant colors indicative of high antioxidant content— dark green leaves, orange/yellow vegetables, purple/blue fruits, and vegetables. Let your meal plate be a rainbow of naturally bright-colored nourishment.

Consume six or more servings of fiber-rich whole grains, legumes (beans), and root vegetables (carrots, beets). Add one or two tablespoons of ground flaxseed to your daily intake via incorporation into recipes or as an ingredient in smoothies.

Maintain protein intake consistent with muscular demands. For the average person that means 15 percent of caloric intake or 0.8 g per kilogram body weight. Athletic people will require more protein. Be sure to include servings of wild cold water ocean fish at least three times weekly.

Tantalize your palate by mastering the art of using fresh herbs and spices to add culinary excitement and adventure to your eating. It is an absolute myth that healthy eating has to be bland and boring. Those who think so just have not explored what is possible with the wide range of natural ingredients readily available in health food stores, groceries, and supermarkets across the nation.

5) Supplement your diet for optimal micro-nutrition by taking:
- A high potency vitamin-mineral supplement.
- Additional antioxidants (critical to the protection of omega-3 fatty acids on cell membranes).
- Multiple antioxidant formula including botanical antioxidants or
  – Vitamin E—400 to 800 International Units (IU) daily.
  – Vitamin C—500 to 1,000 mg daily.

How much omega-3 fatty acids should you take and in what form? As we have seen repeatedly in the medical/scientific literature, adequacy of intake of products of lab-certified purity and potency is fundamental to success.

For vegetarians and others who choose to use flaxseed oil as their omega-3 supplement, the basic dosing recommendation is one tablespoon per 100 pounds of body weight. This approach also allows parents to adjust children's dosing in proportion to body weight. If flaxseed oil is chosen, it is imperative to make food and supplement choices that enhance the activity of enzymes that convert flax's omega-3s into EPA and DHA. This means minimizing the factors that inhibit these enzymes, including reducing trans fats from heated polyunsaturated vegetable oils, omega-6s and intake of alcohol and refined carbohydrates that rapidly elevate insulin levels. Ensure adequate intake of vitamins B_3, B_6, and C, as well as magnesium and zinc to support optimal enzyme activity.

For those who choose fish oil, the recommended maintenance dose is one gram (1,000 mg) of EPA / DHA daily. To address specific health issues, the recommended dose is two to six grams (3,000 to 6,000 mg) daily in divided doses. At these levels, monitoring by a health professional is imperative. Throughout this book, we provide specific ratios of EPA to DHA as well.

TOXICITY, CONTRAINDICATIONS, CAUTIONS, AND INTERACTIONS

Be aware of the following precautions and make your health professional aware of them also.

Ensure adequate intake of a broad range of antioxidants, including vitamin E, to protect the large number of double bonds in ALA, EPA, and DHA from oxidative disruption.

Hypervitaminosis of A and D is possible with abuse of fish liver oils, especially cod liver oil—although Icelandic cod liver oil has had these nutrients reduced purposely to avoid such problems. Pregnant women and women who can become pregnant must be careful about excessive intake of vitamin A due to its birth-defect potential. Fish oils not extracted from liver sources are usually not problematic in this regard. Consult label nutrient listings and manufacturers to ascertain levels of these fat-soluble vitamins.

While decreasing hypertriglyceridemia, fish oils can, in some cases, increase LDL-cholesterol; each patient should be carefully monitored for this idiosyncratic response. This aberrant LDL status can be controlled in hyperlipidemia patients if the fish oil is used in the context of a broad-range natural protocol—including diet improvements, fiber, garlic, pantethine, and inositol hexaniacinate.

Due to their effects on platelet function, fish oil supplements affect bleeding time in a fashion dependent on dosage, duration, and fatty acid composition. In the recommended maintenance dose range, recent studies indicate little if any increase in bleeding time. Nevertheless, it is prudent to monitor bleeding times in pregnant women and patients on anti-coagulant medicines (e.g., aspirin, coumadin) and adjust the pharmaceutical dosage accordingly.

Fish oil can increase homocysteine concentrations and nitric oxide metabolism in healthy humans, with potential effects on vascular integrity.[237] This effect should be monitored and addressed with controlling natural interventions (supplemental folic acid and vitamin B_{12}).

People with either diabetes or schizophrenia may not convert ALA to EPA and DHA efficiently; therefore, people with these conditions should use dietary sources rich in EPA and DHA.

FINAL THOUGHTS

The complete package we are describing here is the kind of program your body will get excited about. It will reward you with increasing vitality and sense of health and well-being.

Appendixes

APPENDIX A

Executive Office of the President

OFFICE OF MANAGEMENT AND BUDGET
WASHINGTON, D.C. 20503
FOR IMMEDIATE RELEASE 2003-13
May 28, 2003

TO SAVE LIVES, OMB URGES REVISING DIETARY GUIDELINES

New information on reducing heart disease risk encouraged

Washington, DC – OMB today urged the Departments of Health and Human Services (HHS) and Agriculture (USDA) to revise the nation's dietary guidelines to include new information that omega-3 fatty acids may reduce the risk of coronary heart disease (CHD), while *trans* fatty acids may increase the risk of CHD. Since CHD kills over 500,000 Americans each year, even a small improvement in dietary habits could save thousands of lives. A copy of the letter sent to HHS and USDA follows this release.

"Health researchers have found that Americans can significantly reduce the risk of heart disease with a modest change in their diets. The government should make this life-saving information as widely available as possible," said Dr. John Graham, Administrator of OMB's Office of Information and Regulatory Affairs (OIRA).

In the letter, OMB recommends that HHS and USDA modify the *Dietary Guidelines and Food Guide Pyramid,* the cornerstones of the government's nutritional information. The Dietary Guidelines affect the content of more than 25 million school lunches, while the *Food Guide Pyramid* appears on many food products, providing consumers with an outline of what to eat each day. Revised every five years, the *Dietary Guidelines* are scheduled to be updated in 2005. *The Food Guide Pyramid* has not been updated since 1992.

According to recent articles in the *American Journal of Clinical Nutrition,* following the current *Dietary Guidelines* only reduces slightly the risk of cardiovascular diseases such as CHD. In the letter, OMB recommends that HHS and USDA take into account new evidence on the benefits of omega-3 fatty acids and risks of *trans* fatty acids when revising the nation's dietary guidelines. For example, the American Heart Association recently revised its dietary guidelines to recommend consuming fish, which is high in omega-3 fatty acids, twice weekly to prevent CHD.

The letter continues the Bush Administration's efforts to help Americans lead longer, better, and healthier lives. The President's 2004 budget proposes a $100 million increase for combating diabetes, reducing rates of obesity, and alleviating the health complications due to asthma. In 2002, the President launched the HealthierUS Initiative, which promotes physical fitness and sports participation among all Americans, with an emphasis on children and adolescents.

OMB's recommendations come in the form of a "prompt" letter, a tool introduced by the Bush Administration. While not forcing agency action, prompt letters alert agencies to issues that OMB considers worthy of priority status. All "prompt" letters, as well as agency responses, can be viewed at *www.omb.gov.* Here is the letter....

May 27, 2003
Honorable Claude A. Allen, Deputy Secretary
Department of Health and Human Services
Washington, D.C. 20201

Honorable James R. Moseley, Deputy Secretary
Department of Agriculture
Washington, D.C. 20250

Dear Mr. Allen and Mr. Moseley:

The purpose of this letter is to request that the Department of Agriculture (USDA) and the Department of Health and Human Services (HHS) further incorporate the large body of recent public health evidence linking food consumption patterns to health and disease as the *Dietary Guidelines for Americans* is revised for its scheduled 2005 release and to update the *Food Guide Pyramid,* which was introduced in 1992.

Secretary Thompson has made it clear that both childhood overweight and adult obesity and the associated chronic health problems such as heart disease are widespread in the United States, and have become one of our nation's most important public health problems. However, recent studies suggest that adherence to the *Dietary Guidelines* has only modest impact on the risk of cardiovascular disease and no significant impact on other chronic diseases such as cancer. OMB believes that these and other studies should play a prominent role as USDA and HHS revise the guidelines. Given the wide reach of the federal nutrition guidelines, we believe that good nutrition habits fostered by improved information on the links between diet and health will have a significant health impact, especially in reducing heart disease. Coronary heart disease (CHD) is our nation's largest cause of premature death for both men and women, killing over 500,000 Americans each year. Even a modest improvement in dietary habits may lead to significant reductions in the number of premature deaths from CHD.

We recognize that the 2000 *Dietary Guidelines* made some changes in recommendations that may reduce cardiovascular risk. We nonetheless urge you to reconsider all available nutritional and medical evidence as you develop the new guidelines. For example, in a previous letter addressed to HHS, we encouraged the Food and Drug Administration (FDA) to finalize a rule to require a product's Nutrition Facts panel to include the amount of *trans* fatty acids present in foods. As you know, there is a growing body of scientific evidence, both experimental and epidemiological, that suggests consumption of trans fatty acids increases the risk of CHD. Another important risk factor is the omega-3 fatty acid content of food. Both epidemiological and clinical studies find that an increase in consumption of omega-3 fatty acids results in reduced deaths due to CHD. The recent revision of the American Heart Association's (AHA's) dietary guidelines recognizes this evidence by recommending consuming fish, which is high in omega-3 fatty acids, at least twice weekly to reduce the risk of CHD. In addition, the AHA recommends the inclusion of oils and other food sources high in omega-3 fatty acids.

The current *Dietary Guidelines* targets only the reduction of saturated fat and cholesterol, with only a brief reference to the risks from trans fatty acids and benefits of omega-3 fatty acids. We encourage you to consider strengthening the language in the guidance and to modify the *Food Guide Pyramid* to better differentiate the health benefits and risks from foods. As noted in the *Report of the Dietary Guidelines Advisory Committee on the Dietary Guidelines for Americans* (2000), consumers find the *Food Guide Pyramid* to be the most useful part of the *Guidelines* and the *Guidelines* itself encourages readers to "let the pyramid guide your food choices." Yet the current *Food Guide Pyramid,* for example, groups meat, poultry, fish, dry beans, eggs, and nuts into a single "Meat and Beans Group" when research suggests that these foods may not be equivalent in terms of their health effects.

Given the significant potential improvement in public health suggested by current evidence, we urge you to consider revising the *Dietary Guidelines* and *Food Guide Pyramid* to emphasize the benefits of reducing foods high in *trans* fatty acids and increasing consumption of foods rich in omega-3 fatty acid.

We would like to set up a meeting with your agencies in the next few weeks to discuss this issue.

As always, the OIRA staff stands ready to assist you in these efforts.

Sincerely,

John D. Graham

Administrator

Office of Information and Regulatory Affairs

APPENDIX B

Resources

We strongly encourage the purchase of quality-oriented, purified, pharmaceutical grade fish oil products. One company that we recommend, Iceland Health, has been producing fish oils since 1938 when Icelander Tryggvi Olafsson and his brother Thordur recognized that modern food processing had created a significant need for vitamins A and D. In the following years, the company became the largest producer of cod liver oil for export to the United States. Between 1938 and 1950, it exported large quantities of its cod liver oil to UpJohn, where the vitamins A and D were extracted.

The production of medicinal cod liver oil for the consumer market started in 1959. Ever since, the Icelandic market has played an essential role as a benchmark, testing ground and research site. The company leads the way in its field and has emphasized quality control as a decisive factor in successfully developing, manufacturing and selling its products. Backed by a worldwide network of contacts and sources for the purchasing, handling and marketing of pharmaceutical grade omega-3 oils and other marine lipids, the company is set to maintain leadership in the future.

With over 60 years of leadership and experience in the production of pure products that improve health and the quality of life, the company is among the world's foremost firms in research, product development, and quality control.

Iceland Health brings to the public these products to new markets efficiently and cost-effectively. Its processing plant is uniquely equipped with the highly specialized production units necessary for complete fish oil processing, including separation of:

- the oil from the fish;
- water and impurities from the oil;
- and valuable components by distillation.

This equipment has been extensively designed to minimize oxidation of the oil and to remove taste and smell in the final product by natural means.

Quality is recognized as the most important factor in the company's business. To implement these principles, management has established a Certified Quality System that conforms to the ISO 9002 international standard. Furthermore, the company has extended the scope of the above standard by incorporating special requirements for sanitary measures, work surroundings and premises. These factors are subject to regulations of Good Manufacturing Practice and Pharmaceutical Production, a prerequisite for obtaining authorization for pharmaceutical production and packaging. It is one of the very few companies producing these products to attain such a high standard. Finally, all products are frequently tested by licensed third party laboratories for potency and purity.

To obtain Iceland Health omega-3 fish oils, cod liver and shark oils, contact the company in the United States:

Iceland Health, Inc.

140 Pike St

Box 1544

Mattituck, NY 11952

(866) 3-ICELAND

Website: www.icelandhealth.com

E-mail: *custserv@icelandhealth.com*

Other brands we recommend that sell pharmaceutical grade fish oil include:

Olde World Icelandic Cod Liver Oil

This product from Garden of Life is another natural, carefully tested cod liver oil. The oil comes from the pure cold waters of Iceland and is cold processed using traditional methods that ensure all of the naturally occurring vitamins and omega-3 essential fatty acids remain intact, while removing any undesirable contaminants.

Other cod liver oils remove the naturally occurring vitamin A and D during the deodorization process and then supplement the finished product with a synthetic form of these vitamins. Garden of Life's Olde World Icelandic Cod Liver Oil is undeodorized, unbleached and contains only the naturally occurring vitamins A and D.

Olde World Icelandic Cod Liver Oil is made with a pleasant tasting all natural lemon-mint flavor to eliminate the fishy aftertaste reminiscent of your grandma's cod liver oil.

Availability—Garden of Life's Olde World Icelandic Cod Liver Oil is available at natural health centers and from health professionals nationwide. For help in finding Garden of Life formulas in your area, contact Garden of Life toll-free at (800) 622-8986 or use the store locator service on their website at *www.gardenoflifeusa.com.*

Icelandic Fish Oil—Worldwide Suppliers

Oriola oy
Orionintie 5,
02200 Espoo
Finland
Tel. 00 358 9 429 99
Fax.00 358 9 429 3031
Tarja.fingerroos@oriola.com

Oriola Vilnius UAB
Laisves pr. 75,
2022 Vilnius
Lithuania
Tel. 00 370 5 2688401
Fax. 00 370 5 2688400

Oriola Estonia
Saku tn. 8
EE0013 Tallinn
Eesti
Estonia
Tel.00372 6 500 710
Fax. 00372 6 500 720

Oriola Latvia
Sencu 4,
Riga, LV-1012
Latvia
Tel. 00371 733 9104
Fax.00371 7802460

P. Lykkeberg A/S
Kattegatvej 75,
DK-2100 Köbenhavn
DANMARK
Tel. 00 45 39 16 92 00
Fax. 00 45 39 16 92 01

EDApharm
Lot C 18-2,
Jalan Ampang Utama 1/1
One Ampang Avenue
6800 Ampang
Selangor Darul Ehsan
Malaysia
Tel. 00 603 4252 2995
Fax. 00 603 4252 3003
edapharm@tm.net.my

MarinEx
Pharmaceuticals Pte
192 Panda Loop 07-18/19
Pantech Industrial Complex
Singapore 128381

Vermer S.A.R.L
7 Rue Rosa Bonheur
750 15 Paris
France
Fax. 0033 15658 0125

Island Export-Import
Chwarznienska Str. 192C
Gdynia
Polland
Tel. 00 48 58 624 91 51;
00 48 58 624 91 57
Fax. 00 48 58 624 91 57
island@pro.onet.pl

Cansin—Medikal Ilaç San.
Tic. Ltd. Sti.
Suleyman Sirri Sokak No:
16/5 Sihhiye
ANKARA
Turkey
Tel. 00 90 312 433 7424
Fax. 00 90 312 431 29 97

ZEST Co. Ltd.
Chingeltei District
33A-31 Khoroo VI
Ulaanbaatar
Mongolia
Tel. 00 976 11 318 796
zestxxk@yahoo.com

Ágúst KárasonTaiwan
23-3, 2f, Touliao
9 Lin, Fuan Li, Dashi Cheng
335
Taoyuan Shien
TAIWAN
Tel. 03-3880019;
gsm 0927-504149
agustkara@softhome.net;
agust@northtrade.cc

SC Cons.Energdon Aldis
SRL
STR. Podgoria nr 2B
JUD. BIHOR
3700 ORADEA
RUMENIA
Fax. 0040 259 433305

Wild Salmon

Barlean's Fishery
4936 Lake Terrell Road
Ferndale WA 98248
360 384 0325

The best canned wild salmon, rich in omega-3s and ecologically harvested, in the country.

Prescription Pain Relievers vs. Fish Oils for Osteoarthritis

If you have read this far, you know that inflammation is a serious underlying factor in many of the illnesses that rob Americans of energy, zest for life, good health and—sometimes—of life itself. At the very least, chronic inflammation ages the body more quickly, both outside and in. A slow burn of inflammation is an implicated factor in heart disease, cancer, arthritis (primarily rheumatoid, and sometimes in advanced osteoarthritis), and Alzheimer's disease. You also know that the imbalance of omega-3 oils to omega-6 oils that exists in virtually every American's body powerfully contributes to a state of chronic inflammation.

Drugs have been used to try to rein in inflammation—and the pain that often comes with it—since the late 1800s, when aspirin was first developed. Since that time, several different classes of drugs designed to relieve inflammation and pain and to reduce fever have been developed. As a group, all of these drugs are known as *nonsteroidal anti-inflammatory drugs*, or NSAIDs. They were so named because they reduce pain and inflammation just as steroid drugs do, but through a completely different biochemical mode of action.

Long before the advent of pharmaceutical technology, humans used whole plants or parts of plants for this same purpose. White willow bark, the substance from which aspirin was first derived, was once chewed as a remedy for pain. Ginger, turmeric, and green tea are other natural anti-inflammatories that have been used the world over for millennia to support balanced health. Herbs and other plants have long been utilized to help relieve fever and pain.

With all we know now about the anti-inflammatory effects of omega-3 oils, it makes perfect sense to use them for these purposes. Current research demonstrates that they modulate inflammation in many of the same ways the NSAIDs do. Because of the way these fats enhance the health of multiple body systems, they do not carry the same risks as the NSAIDs—risks that have proven to be a nagging and significant concern.

It is accepted fact that NSAIDs do not have any effect on the course of a disease process; they do not effect a cure or improve the underlying disease that is causing the inflammation. Since the imbalance of omega-6 to omega-3 is so often an important cause of inflammation, supplying the body with adequate omega-3 while reducing omega-6 intake could very well take the place of these drugs—particularly the newest members of the class, the COX-2 drugs: Vioxx (rofecoxib), Bextra (valdecoxib), and Celebrex (celecoxib).

The promise of the COX-2 inhibitor drugs seemed enormous. In large trials of these drugs as arthritis and pain therapies, an unexpected benefit kept coming up: Risk of developing or dying from some cancers was less for the patients on the COX-2 inhibitors. It also became apparent that Alzheimer's disease risk fell with long-term COX-2 therapy. These results were so consistent that many studies were instituted to examine the potential of these drugs for the prevention of these feared diseases—among them, the studies of Vioxx and Celebrex that led to the first being removed from the market and the other's safety being seriously questioned.

THE STORY OF VIOXX

At the end of September 2004, the pain medicine Vioxx (rofecoxib) was voluntarily withdrawn by Merck & Co. The drug had been heavily promoted as a "super-aspirin" since it hit the market in 2000, prescribed primarily for the relief of pain caused by osteoarthritis. It had been prescribed to millions of people and earned its maker $2.5 billion worldwide in the year 2003 alone, and made over a billion dollars in 2004 before it was withdrawn. Why? Because at least two large studies had pointed to a major flaw of this blockbuster drug: increased risk of heart attacks and stroke.

The study that nailed the lid onto Vioxx's coffin was the APPROVe (Adenomatous Polyp Prevention on Vioxx) trial.[238] In it, approximately 2,600 subjects with a history of colorectal polyps (a precancerous condition) were given one of a range of dosages of Vioxx or placebo. Before the study was over, it became evident to the researchers that taking over 25 mg per day of Vioxx for over 18 months *tripled* the risk of heart attack or stroke. Patients taking less than 25 mg per day showed a less dramatic increase in risk, but a trend towards higher risk of circulatory problems persisted.

Earlier trials had pointed in this same direction.[239] In 2000, the VIGOR (Vioxx Gastrointestinal Outcomes Research) trial was performed to compare the gastrointestinal safety of Vioxx to that of an older pain medicine, naproxen. Vioxx came out on top with regards to GI safety, but it increased the risk of cardiovascular events. These results prompted the FDA to demand warnings on Vioxx's labeling about the potential for increased risk of heart attack and stroke while on these drugs—warnings that, in the end, went largely unnoticed. Merck pushed the drug more strongly than ever, spending an incredible $161 million on direct-to-consumer advertisements for Vioxx in the year 2000.

Many leading health experts—including Eric Topol, M.D., of the Cleveland Clinic; Thomas Moore, a well-known health policy analyst; and even David Graham, the associate director for Science and Medicine at the FDA's Office of Drug Safety—agree that this drug should have been withdrawn years before Merck pulled the plug.[240]

CELEBREX IS FAIR GAME, TOO

Concerns are also being raised about Celebrex in the wake of drastic increases in heart attack and stroke risk during a trial of high doses of the drug for prevention of colon polyps. This top-selling arthritis drug, prescribed to 27 million Americans, was found to raise heart attack and stroke risk by two and a half times (at a dose of 400 mg per day) to 3.4 times (at a dose of 800 mg per day). These troubling findings were released just 11 weeks following the withdrawal of Vioxx. Drug company stocks went tumbling, and doctors began to think twice before writing a prescription for any of the drugs in this class. Over 40 studies funded by the National Institutes of Health—studies investigating the use of COX-2 inhibition for the prevention and treatment of cancer, Alzheimer's disease, and other diseases—were suspended pending an FDA review of this class of medications.

ONLY A BIG LOSS FOR BIG PHARMA

After all the hype, the sad truth is that these drugs weren't a notable improvement over much older, much cheaper drugs. This fact is obvious to anyone who delves into the actual research on the COX-2 inhibitor drugs—a class that includes Vioxx, Celebrex (celecoxib), and Bextra (valdecoxib)—in comparison with older drugs for pain and inflammation. Dr. John Abramson may have said it best, during an interview on CNN: "Patients need to know that giving up Celebrex does not mean they are giving up the best drug."

European researchers recently released a report showing that these drugs are actually of limited use in relieving pain. In a review of 23 previous clinical trials published in the *British Medical Journal*, COX-2 drugs were found to be, in the short term, only slightly superior to placebo. In the long term, the drugs showed no advantage over placebo. When asked about the results of his study, lead researcher Jan Magnus Bjordal, M.D., stated that he and the other researchers "were surprised that the effects were so small. Given the serious adverse effects that the drugs can cause, doctors need...to review carefully whether their use...[is] justified."[241]

Studies on the effect of COX-2 drugs on cancer and Alzheimer's risk, despite revelations of excess risks to the heart, were promising. The trend in those studies confirmed that COX-2 is involved in the progression of some cancers and possibly in Alzheimer's disease progression, and that minimizing its activity could well be an important part of preventing and treating these diseases. Unfortunately, it looks as though long-term use of these drugs in appropriate dosages would pose too great a danger to circulatory health to merit their use for disease prevention in healthy people.

The COX-2 story hasn't yet ended, however. We now know that many natural substances, including fish oils, downregulate COX-2 activity. They don't do so as selectively as do the drugs, but this is not a bad thing. Think of omega-3 oils as a natural balancer of COX activity: They balance prostaglandin production in the way Nature intended. And, as an extra bonus, we know that omega-3 oils are extraordinarily heart-healthy. There's not a chance that they could raise risk of heart disease like Vioxx.

What went wrong? How could the fruit of the labors of so many brilliant scientific minds—the COX-2 drugs, which were thoroughly reviewed by the FDA, approved, aggressively marketed and promoted, and prescribed to millions of people—turn out to be such a bust? And can fish oils really substitute for these drugs in people with osteoarthritis and rheumatoid arthritis?

Let's understand this by first explaining how NSAIDs work, and how the COX-2 drugs were supposed to be a big improvement (and weren't). Then, we will tell you why proper fatty acid nutrition can relieve pain, stiffness, and inflammation in the joints—and how current scientific evidence indicates that omega-3 fatty acid supplementation may, in fact, slow or reverse the biochemical processes that degrade cartilage in osteoarthritis.

NSAIDs AND COX ENZYMES

The COX (cyclooxygenase) enzymes are ubiquitous—they are found in virtually every cell of the human body. Two forms of the enzyme exist: COX-1 and COX-2. The job of the COX enzymes is to transform the omega-6 fatty acid *arachidonic acid* (AA) into prostaglandins.

The COX-1 enzyme is responsible for the production of so-called "housekeeping" prostaglandins that maintain the integrity of the gastrointestinal lining, support kidney function, and participate in hormone activity. COX-1 activity also promotes *platelet aggregation*, the clumping together of blood platelets that can, in excess, thicken blood and increase risk of occlusive heart attacks and strokes.

The COX-2 enzyme is somewhat more sinister; it is found in 20-fold heightened concentrations in body cells that are inflamed. It pushes the inflammatory response into high gear, leading to the production of multiple prostaglandins and growth factors that accelerate inflammation and tissue degeneration. Unrelenting chronic inflammation is now known to increase the risk of some cancers, as well.

Drugs of the NSAID class relieve pain and inflammation by blocking the action of COX enzymes. The older NSAIDs (aspirin, diflunisal, disalcid, trilisate, diclofenac, alclofenac, fenclofenac, tolmetin, etodolac, indomethacin, sulindac, oxaprozin, drugs ending in –profen, drugs ending in –icam, nabumetone) block both the COX-1 and COX-2 enzymes to varying degrees. The COX-2 inhibitor drugs (valdecoxib, celecoxib, rofecoxib), as you might guess, selectively inhibit COX-2.

Both the older NSAIDs and the COX-2 inhibitors relieve pain and reduce inflammation. This is why both types of drug are used extensively to treat osteoarthritis and rheumatoid arthritis. Although osteoarthritis rarely involves true inflammation—which is characterized by swelling, redness, heat, and pain—NSAIDs still work to reduce discomfort caused by cartilage deterioration by blocking the formation of prostaglandins that amplify and transmit pain signals within the body.

The older NSAIDs also reduce platelet aggregation by blocking COX-1 activity—which explains why aspirin is so useful for the prevention of heart disease. Unfortunately, the older generation of NSAIDs also block the helpful effects of COX-1 in the gastrointestinal tract. GI bleeding is common in those who use these NSAIDs long term—a side effect that, according to the *New England Journal of Medicine*, is the cause of over 100,000 hospitalizations and 16,500 deaths per year.[242] The blood-thinning effect of the drug further increased this risk, delaying the sealing shut of the GI ulceration and prolonging bleeding time.

To counter this problem, drug researchers looked for a way to selectively inhibit the COX-2 enzyme. They did, and Vioxx, Celebrex, and Bextra were born. Early on in the life history of these drugs, researchers suspected that there might be an increased risk of heart attack or stroke because of the lack of COX-1 effect. Large-scale studies began to confirm this suspicion by 2001. Vioxx is 1,000 times more selective for COX-2 than older NSAIDs; Celebrex is only 375 times more selective than the older drugs. It appears that maximal COX-2 selectivity is not a good thing.

These new, supposedly improved drugs for pain and inflammation lowered one risk of NSAIDs (GI bleeding), but in doing so they increased another risk (cardiovascular events) so much that risk surpassed benefit.

RAMPANT PRESCRIPTION DRUG DANGERS

Motivation to turn to less risky natural alternatives to prescription drugs is greater than ever before. New news stories about prescription drug risks are everywhere.

According to a story published in the *New York Times* in mid-December of 2004, "[t]he $500 billion drug company dynasty finally appears ready to fall as the industry struggles to save face among continual reports of serious problems with well-known drugs."

The problems go beyond simple mistakes on the part of drug makers. Investigative journalists have uncovered a pattern of denial and subterfuge that kept Vioxx on the market too long.[243] This pattern involved Merck, the scientists Merck hired to crank out positive research on the drug, and the FDA, an organization that many experts claim should have taken more aggressive steps to protect consumers as soon as the first studies pointed to increased cardiovascular risk in 2001.

Patterns of deception have been found in marketing, promotion, and FDA approval of several other drugs, including the diabetes drug Rezulin, hormone replacement drug PremPro, and several of the popular SSRI antidepressants.

More bad news for Big Pharma:

* The massively popular class of antidepressant drugs known as SSRIs (selective serotonin reuptake inhibitors), once regarded as totally safe, has been raked over the coals in recent months because of evidence that they increase the risk of suicidal and violent behavior in children and adults.

* Eli Lilly recently warned that Strattera, its newest ADHD drug, could cause severe liver injury.

* Rezulin, a drug that was once prescribed for type 2 diabetes, was found to drastically increase risk of liver failure. Dozens of people died from liver failure related to its use before the drug was pulled from the market.

* Cholesterol-lowering drug Baycol was also withdrawn when it became evident that it was harmful—potentially deadly—because of the damage it can cause to the liver.

* Remicade, a drug prescribed for rheumatoid arthritis and Crohn's disease (a chronic inflammatory condition that afflicts the large intestine) was linked, in 2004, with potentially fatal blood disorders and disorders of the central nervous system. Of roughly 509,000 patients who have taken Remicade, 580 have reported significant or serious adverse effects.

In the pages of this book, we have given detailed explanations of how proper omega-3 nutrition can at least partially replace drugs for the treatment of all of these conditions. Osteoarthritis and rheumatoid arthritis are no exceptions.

Let's look specifically at how omega-3 fats support better joint health—while, contrary to the heart-threatening effects of the COX-2 inhibitor drugs, they improve cardiovascular health in several important ways. In fact, we would argue that omega-3 fats are Nature's most potent defense against heart attack and stroke.

OMEGA-3 OILS AND OSTEOARTHRITIS

Many more research studies have examined the effects of fish oils on rheumatoid arthritis than on osteoarthritis. As you learned in Chapter 8, RA is a disease of excessive inflammation, and the mechanism by which omega-3s defuse excessive inflammation is well understood. The role of omega-3s, such as DHA, EPA, and ALA, in reducing pain and cartilage deterioration in osteoarthritis—a condition that rarely can be characterized as inflammatory—is less well understood. Research has shown that they do help relieve osteoarthritis pain and stiffness, however, and our understanding of exactly why this is grows by the year. What that research shows is that omega-3 supplementation appears to actually inhibit, or even reverse, the process of cartilage degeneration that is osteoarthritis. A sampling of the current research:

- In one study published in the *Journal of Biological Chemistry* in January 2000, researchers found that the incorporation of omega-3 fats—but not of other fats—into articular cartilage chondrocyte membranes (translation: the membranes of cartilage cells) resulted in decreased activity of cartilage-degrading enzymes and in the expression of inflammatory cytokines, as well as COX-2.[244] The omega-3s did *not* affect COX-1.

- A study from the same group of researchers, based at the Connective Tissue Biology Laboratories at the Cardiff School of Biosciences in England, was published in the journal *Arthritis and Rheumatism* in June of 2002. The study's aim was to determine whether omega-3 supplementation would affect the metabolism of osteoarthritic cartilage. They found that adding omega-3s to osteoarthritic cartilage "abolished the expression of mRNA for mediators of inflammation (cyclooxygenase 2, 5-lipoxygenase, tumor necrosis factor alpha…IL-1 alpha, and IL-1 beta) without affecting the expression…[of] several other proteins involved in normal tissue homeostasis." In other words, the tissue markers of OA can be significantly altered—for the better—by the addition of omega-3 fats. The research team added some other types of fats to some of their samples, and found no such benefit.[245]

- In yet another study by the Cardiff group—this one, published in February of 2004—patients undergoing joint replacement for the treatment of osteoarthritis were given either cod liver oil or placebo. Cartilage samples were analyzed after surgery, and these samples showed that 86 percent of the patients who took cod liver oil had significantly lowered or absent levels of enzymes that cause cartilage damage. Only 26 percent of the placebo patients had lowered or absent levels of these enzymes. In the cod liver oil group, there was also a marked decrease in some of the enzymes that cause joint pain.[246]

- In 1989, the journal *Lancet* published a letter from a research group who gave 10 mls per day of EPA (in the form of the fish oil MaxEPA) or placebo (olive oil) to 26 OA patients. Every day of each fourth week, the patients assessed their pain and degree of interference of their arthritis in their daily activities. After six months of therapy, the patients on cod liver oil showed less pain and less interference with daily activities. The difference was not statistically significant, however. (This means that, according to statistical analysis, it is possible that the patients on cod liver oil showed greater improvement only due to chance, rather than because of the effects of the supplement.)

- In a poster presentation at the Third International Conference on Essential Fatty Acids and Eicosanoids in Adelaide, Australia, researchers presented a paper on cartilage deterioration, aging, osteoarthritis, and levels of omega-6 fats in cartilage. They had evaluated fatty acid status of cartilage samples taken from autopsies or from surgical procedures, across a range of ages and disease states. It was found that the cartilage of younger subjects was relatively deficient in omega-6 fats and higher in an omega-3 fatty acid called Mead acid (eicosatrienoic acid; this fat is made from other omega-3s in the body and is found mostly in connective tissue, and is also found in fish oils). Samples from older individuals had higher levels of omega-6 and lower Mead acid; samples from weight-bearing joints such as the hips or spine had higher omega-6 levels than non-weight-bearing joints and even lower Mead acid, suggesting a relationship between wear and tear and heightened omega-6 levels. Finally, cartilage that was osteoarthritic had the highest omega-6 and lowest Mead acid levels of all. The authors conclude that "accumulation of omega-6 EFAs in cartilage might predispose towards the development of OA, and that the presence of Mead acid might somehow be protective."[247]

- A 2002 test-tube study found that cartilage degradation in samples from osteoarthritic human and cow joints was significantly slowed with addition of omega-3s to the mix. This protective effect was not found with addition of omega-6 fats. The techniques used in this study are accepted in the scientific community as an excellent model of the arthritic process, and allowed the research team to demonstrate that omega-3s from fish oil decrease both degradative and inflammatory aspects of osteoarthritic changes in cartilage cells—with no adverse effects on normal, healthy tissues.[248]

We also know from the research that eicosapentaenoic acid (EPA) has a stimulatory effect on collagen synthesis, the process that creates new cartilage. The conversion of the omega-6 fat arachidonic acid into prostaglandin E2 (PGE2), however, has cartilage-degrading effects, increasing the activity and production of biochemicals in the body that cause inflammation and cartilage breakdown, and possibly leading to joint inflammation and pain.[249]

The research into omega-3s for osteoarthritis is still young. Further studies are needed to discern what dosage schedule and concentration of DHA and/or EPA will prove most helpful. At this writing, however, the risks of omega-3 supplementation are so low and the potential for benefit so great that osteoarthritis patients can certainly give them a try—either instead of or in conjunction with NSAID therapy. (Do not stop taking your usual medications without a doctor's guidance.)

FISH OILS AND RHEUMATOID ARTHRITIS

The benefits of omega-3 fats from fish oil for rheumatoid arthritis patients are well established.[250] EPA is most helpful, and has been found to reduce multiple markers of joint inflammation and degradation in numerous studies. Arachidonic acid metabolites (the pro-inflammatory prostaglandins and leukotrienes) are known to exacerbate every aspect of rheumatoid arthritis, and omega-3 fats and their metabolites have been demonstrated to antagonize these pathological processes. Significant improvements in joint tenderness and morning stiffness have been seen in multiple published trials of fish oil supplementation for this potentially debilitating illness.[251]

If you are an RA patient, you may be wondering why no one on your medical team has clued you in on the benefits of fish oil for your disease. The sad truth is that fish oils, being natural substances, cannot be patented by drug companies. Without patent protection, the drug makers can't make the kind of money they make on patentable, synthetic drugs. Drug company marketing is physicians' main source of information on valuable therapies, and drug companies aren't sending their reps out to tell rheumatologists about the value of fish oil.

ALL THIS—AND IMPROVED HEART HEALTH, TOO

Using fish oils to help relieve arthritis symptoms won't increase your heart disease risk like COX-2 inhibitor drugs do. Here's a brief review of the effect of omega-3s on heart health. Omega-3s:

- are incorporated into the lining of arteries, enhancing their flexibility and protecting against "hardening of the arteries";
- increase "good" HDL and decrease "bad" LDL cholesterol;

- lower triglycerides, a major heart disease risk factor, better than any other natural compound;
- decrease levels of C-reactive protein, a marker of inflammation in the arteries, now known to be a heart disease risk marker as important as cholesterol;
- decrease fibrinogen, which converts to fibrin, a major component of blood clots;
- reduce lipoprotein(a), a lipid fraction that is also a marker of heart disease risk;
- counter the pro-inflammatory effects of omega-6 and trans fats in both circulatory system and joints;
- lower blood pressure (at high doses);
- reduce risk of heart arrhythmias (irregular heart rhythms) and sudden death related to arrhythmia.

LOOK TO NATURE FOR JOINT HEALING

Natural substances—herbs, vitamins, minerals, and plant chemicals (phytochemicals) derived from herbs and foods—are not highly specific. They are not "magic bullets." They work in a broader, more comprehensive fashion than pharmaceuticals, in cooperation with the natural workings of the human body. This is why side effects are so much more rare than with pharmaceuticals. When they do occur, they are mild, and in many instances, they move the body in the direction of improved health. Omega-3 fats improve the functioning of more than one body system. In fact, it's hard to think of any body system that *doesn't* benefit when better omega-3/omega-6 balance is reached.

Many doctors remain ignorant about its usefulness in osteoarthritis, rheumatoid arthritis, and other conditions. You may be the first to let your doctor know that this therapy is of proven benefit!

The Beauty of Omega-3

Most beauty regimens focus on the outside of the body, with skin creams, lotions, serums and treatments leading the way and promising beautiful skin, tough nails and even glorious hair. However, essential fatty acids like omega-3 are fast giving rise to a new kind of beauty treatment, one that works from the inside out.

The body has chemical messengers known as prostaglandins, which strongly influence external health. They are not stored in the body but must be constantly synthesized from essential fatty acids that come from the diet and are deposited in cell membranes. When the body lacks essential fatty acids an imbalance in prostaglandins results, leading to skin, nail and hair problems.

Essential fatty acid deficiency also leads to an imbalance in the levels of hormone-like compounds called eicosanoids. Eicosanoid imbalance may lead to specific skin problems, such as itching, eczema and reddish or dry patches of skin, particularly on the face, arms, legs and buttocks. Essential fatty acid deficiency may also lead to discoloration of the hair, and cracked, broken nails. By increasing the intake of essential fatty acids, either from foods rich in omega-3 like fish, certain grains and nuts as well as flaxseed, or from supplements, we can also increase better internal hydration. Better internal hydration can lead to smoother skin, strong nails and vibrant hair. In other words, omega-3 essential fatty acids are truly beautiful when it comes to beauty.

If we look at each area individually, we'll begin to see just how beautiful they are.

DRY SKIN

Dry skin is often a sign that the body isn't getting enough good fats. Skin cells incorporate essential fatty acids into their membranes, helping to maintain cell structure and function. Healthy cell membranes prevent moisture loss from the skin, help nutrients enter the cell, and prevent toxins from penetrating the cell. Healthy cells are the foundation for beautiful skin.

Understanding the beauty of the skin starts with understanding the structure of its three layers: the epidermis, dermis, and subcutaneous tissue.

The epidermis is the outer layer of skin. Its thickness varies in different types of skin as well as at different parts of the body. It is thinnest on the eyelids at .05 mm and thickest on the palms and soles at 1.5 mm. The epidermis contains five layers: stratum basale, stratum spinosum, stratum granulosum, stratum licidum, and stratum corneum.

The dermis also varies in thickness depending on the location of the skin. It is .3 mm on the eyelid and 3.0 mm on the back. The dermis is composed of three types of tissue that are present throughout: collagen, elastic tissue, and reticular fibers.

The third layer is the subcutaneous tissue, a layer of fat and connective tissue that houses larger blood vessels and nerves. This layer is important in the regulation of temperature of the skin itself as well as the body. It is this layer that feeds on essential fatty acids.

DANDRUFF

The itching and scalp inflammation associated with dandruff may be helped by omega-3 consumption. More importantly, essential fatty acids may go directly to the cause of dandruff, working to slow the rate at which the dry scalp cells slough off and controlling the rate the old cells are replaced by new, healthier, more hydrated cells. All of which leads to a less itchy scalp, less flaking and less fear of wearing black.

ECZEMA

Studies published in the *Journal of International Medical Research* and the *British Journal of Dermatology* report that essential fatty acids can help dramatically reduce the itchy, ugly, symptoms of eczema. Nearly seven percent of the population suffers from skin conditions, such as eczema. Another two to four percent suffer from psoriasis, which is characterized by sharply bordered reddened plaques covered with overlapping silvery scales.

The beauty-enhancing oils from omega-3 fatty acids and other oils (such as borage and evening primrose) are critical to the vitality and youthfulness of skin. In fact, there has even been speculation that a topical application of essential fatty acids, in oils or creams, may work even better. We'll get to that later.

NAILS

Dry, brittle, peeling nails are a sign of something amiss in the diet. Chances are what's missing is essential fatty acids. By increasing the intake of omega-3, we can increase the level of internal hydration and thus increase the strength in finger and toenails.

The fingernail is made of keratin. It acts as a protective plate and enhances sensation of the fingertip. The protective function of the fingernail is commonly known, but the sensation function is equally important. The fingertip has many nerve endings in it allowing us to receive volumes of information about objects we touch. The nail acts as a counterforce to the fingertip, providing even more sensory input when an object is touched.

Nails grow all the time, but their rate of growth slows down with age, poor circulation and poor nutrition. Fingernails grow faster than toenails, at a rate of 3 mm per month. It takes six months for a nail to grow from the root to the free edge. Toenails grow about 1 mm per month and take 12-18 months to be completely replaced.

The structure of the nail is divided into six specific parts: the root, nail bed, nail plate, eponychium (cuticle), perionychium, and hyponychium.

HAIR

Hair has no nerve endings, making it doubly surprising that it reacts so strongly, in essence feeling the lack of moisture at the root. Hair is fed from the root, where vital nutrients infuse the cortex with what's needed for external gloss and internal strength. When hair breaks or splits, it is not getting enough of what it needs. Similarly, when hair is suffering, it acts much like a piece of fabric left too long in the sun. The color fades. Essential fatty acids work from within the cellular structure of the hair follicle (or root), growing with the hair to give a greater sense of shine, smoother surface texture and even solidifying natural color pigmentation.

Hair has two separate structures: the follicle inside the skin and the shaft, the hair we can see.

The follicle is a stocking-like structure that contains several layers with different jobs. At the base of the follicle is a projection called a papilla and it contains capillaries, or tiny blood vessels, that feed the cells. The living part of the hair is the bottom part of the papilla called the bulb. This bottom part is the only part fed by the capillaries. The cells in the bulb divide every 23 to 72 hours, faster than any other cells in the body.

Much has been written about the internal benefits of omega-3, the essential fatty acid that gives fat a good name. Perhaps it's no wonder then that the miracle of this particular fatty acid may extend to external beauty as well, affecting the surface and texture of skin, the health and strength of nails, and even the luster of hair. When coupled with the effect omega-3 can have on the heart, blood flow and other internal organs, this miracle with the science-fiction sounding name may turn out to be one of the easiest and best things a person can do to feel—and look—better from the inside out.

First, a primer on the essentials.

THE ESSENTIAL OMEGA-3

The essence of essential fats goes back to 1929, when the husband-wife research team of George and Mildred Burr discovered that a lack of essential fats in the diet of animals created skin problems, such as dryness and some inflammation. They also observed damage to internal organs that, when left untreated, led to organ failure and ultimately death.

In 1956, another researcher by the name of Hugh Sinclair claimed that most of the world's civilized diseases—among them coronary heart disease, cancer, diabetes, inflammation, strokes and skin disease—were caused by a disturbance in fat metabolism. He theorized that one of the major reasons that life expectancy hadn't changed (at that time) since the middle of the nineteenth century was because the typical Western diet was full of processed foods, saturated fats and other bad fats while lacking sufficient good fats. Not much has changed other than we now know that essential fatty acids like omega-3s have a profoundly positive influence on the body, both internally and, as we're just now discovering, externally.

Recent health trends have taken us toward a more fat-free diet, but it's important to understand that some fat is actually essential to overall health and well-being. In fact, the body needs essential fatty acids just like it needs other essential vitamins and minerals to help prevent and treat numerous diseases. They also help to control a large number of cellular processes.

Physiologically speaking, there are two fatty acids that are truly essential, even though the body cannot manufacture them itself: linoleic acid (LA) and alpha-linolenic acid (ALA), an omega-3 fatty acid. A healthy body uses LA and ALA to produce other fatty acids, which, in turn, produce a host of beneficial compounds, previously mentioned and called eicosanoids. Each play specific roles in maintaining good health, and are known as derivative fatty acids. They include: eicosapentaenoic acid (EPA) and docosahexaenoic acid (DHA), both omega-3 fatty acids.

Many Americans get an excess of linoleic acid from processed foods, margarine and vegetable oils. We get very little of the omega-3s, ALA, EPA and DHA. To change this, the diet must change.

- Eat less processed food, margarine and vegetable oils.
- Eat less fatty red meats, deep fried foods, butter and whole milk.
- Eat more fatty fish like salmon, mackerel, sardines and tuna.

Supplementation may also help since it combines all the essential fatty acids in one convenient capsule. Good supplements of essential fatty acids include flaxseed oil and fish oil. All of these are essential in creating an external environment for beautiful skin.

OMEGA-3s AND THE SKIN

With us from birth, the skin is also an organ essential for life, and one that we tend to abuse as we grow and age. This living, breathing body suit can be the ultimate fashion statement, walking the runway walk and shouting quietly about its health. Treat it kindly and it responds with smooth, glowing affection; treat it harshly, and it responds with dryness, sagging in places that are unseemly, facial lines, uneven pigmentation and other atrocities. As something that literally covers us from head to toe, skin can feel the light touch of a hand, or the harsh heat of fire. It bruises as easily as a broken heart, and it must be cared for. And yet, we don't treat it as joyously as we might. Our neglect leads to dryness, lack of elasticity and more. Sometimes a better diet, more exercise and definitely more water will help, as will as uptake of omega-3.

The two major sources of omega-3 fatty acids are fish, including organic salmon, trout and albacore tuna, and flaxseed. Flaxseed is loaded with alpha-linolenic acid, the brain of the omega-3 fatty acid molecule that assists in maximizing the benefits of nutritious foods. Most foods have far less omega-3 properties than what is found in flaxseed. In fact, one of the foods that many turn to in order to increase their omega-3 dietary intake is nuts. However, as an example, it would take nearly 25 cups of peanut butter to achieve the levels of alpha-linolenic acid found in just 1/4 cup of ground flaxseed. Think of the calorie intake, let alone the stares you might receive while waiting in line at the natural foods store with a cart full of peanut butter, and you'll probably opt for the flaxseed. Or even better, 100 percent natural fish oil. It is believed that the body only converts a small percentage of ALA to EPA and DHA. The omega-3 in fish is already the right structure of bonds to be immediately available as EPA and DHA, thus being a far superior source of omega-3, when ingested, than flaxseed.

Just as an inadequate intake of omega-3 can lead to dry skin, eczema, dermatitis and even premature wrinkling, an adequate intake might help to improve and maintain the smooth texture and natural radiance of skin.

FREE RADICALS COST SKIN ITS YOUTH

When looking for one of the main culprits of worsening skin conditions, look no further than the dreaded free radicals. Free radicals attack the cell membranes of skin cells resulting in the production of toxic inflammatory chemicals. As the skin fights the effects of free radicals, these chemicals trigger the inflammation response of the skin cells that in turn cause the body to produce still more chemicals that digest collagen. Collagen, of course, is the elastic protein band inside skin that keeps it supple and able to spring back into place. Once collagen is digested, micro-scars result and wrinkles appear.

Antioxidants are a great way to help prevent this oxidation-leading-to-wrinkles process. Some of the most commonly recognized antioxidants include vitamins C and E as well as beta-carotene. Another effective response would be to slow the process of skin aging by reducing the inflammatory response of the body. This can be accomplished with proper levels of omega-3.

In addition to protecting our heart and other internal organs, omega-3, especially that consumed from fish, can help lessen the skin's inflammatory response to the toxic chemicals released because of the free radicals. Essentially, the omega-3s stimulate the body to produce anti-inflammatory chemicals instead, thus preventing the eventual breakdown of collagen and so encouraging younger-looking skin.

OMEGA-3 AND INFLAMMATION

Noted dermatologist Nicholas V. Perricone, M.D., has noted the importance of omega-3 fatty acids, obtained from fatty fish, as an important ingredient in natural skin care achieved from the inside out. He is convinced that the deficiency of omega-3s in the diet can lead to premature aging and recommends a diet rich in antioxidants, such as blueberries, strawberries, cranberries and raspberries, in addition to fish rich in omega-3. He also recommends a low-carbohydrate and low-sugar diet because: "Inflammation is triggered by what we eat and anything that is sugar or rapidly converted to sugar (carbohydrates, such as white rice, white breads or pasta) can attach to collagen and cause stiffness of skin or very old-looking skin."[252]

The most important scientific theory behind Perricone's work suggests that aging, with its wrinkles, lines, puffiness and sagging, as well as all diseases ranging from cancer to strokes, are caused by inflammation at the cellular level. He theorizes that by reducing inflammation with the use of powerful antioxidants and anti-inflammatories, it is possible to prevent the signs of aging.

It begins with a nutritional face-lift that uses both antioxidant- and essential fatty acid-rich foods to help reduce inflammation, thus achieving beautiful, glowing skin and vibrant health. By exploring the connection between inflammation, aging and disease on a cellular level, we are able to see aging as a chronic progression caused by free radicals. Controlling free radicals then controls the rate at which we age.

Supplements can help to reduce inflammation and rebuild and rejuvenate the body. Perricone has also detailed the types of vitamins, minerals and amino acids needed to protect collagen from free radical damage, increase metabolic efficiency and strengthen the immune system. They include the aforementioned usual suspects: vitamins C and E.

Exercise also comes into play. In fact, research has shown that flexibility, cardiovascular and strength/endurance training can all have positive anti-inflammatory effects on the body, internally and externally.

In essence, inflammation is at the basis of age-related diseases like heart disease, diabetes, cancer, autoimmune disease, and, now, aged, wrinkled skin. The wrong foods, such as sugar, processed foods, pasta, breads, pastry and baked goods, can increase levels of pro-inflammatory peptides.

Sugar is the number-one enemy, causing inflammation that destroys our bodies and attaches to collagen, which results in hardened, inflexible, and sagging skin. Controlling our blood sugar level and insulin levels will help improve our health as well as present us with potentially beautiful, youthful skin.

An anti-inflammatory diet consists of high-quality protein like that found in fish, colorful fresh fruits and dark leafy-green vegetables, and adequate amounts of good fat like that found in salmon, flax, nuts, seeds and olive oil.

Our skin is a perfect reflection of our internal health, and when skin visibly improves from this anti-inflammatory lifestyle, we automatically reduce our risk of age-related disease. As an added benefit, it is also possible that body weight will normalize, another factor key in caring for skin and promoting external beauty.

In short, omega-3 essential fatty acids are necessary for a healthy immune system, increased mental clarity, normalizing weight (eat fat to burn fat) and beauty that can be seen.

LET THE SUN IN

Omega-3 essential fatty acids may also help prevent sun damage. The link between sun, skin cancer and premature aging is well documented and well publicized. Even so, there are still a number of people who like the look of suntanned skin, finding it cosmetically desirable. Witness the rise of fake-tanning creams and lotions.

Sunscreen manufacturers now include high sun protection factors (SPFs) in their creams and oils, with some claiming to have an SPF of 50 or higher. Most fall into the 15 to 20 range. But oil on the body is not the only defense against the sun's harmful rays; oil in the body can also help protect against sunburn and perhaps even help prevent skin cancer.

One of the many health benefits of omega-3s also appears to be internal protection against the external sun. It functions much like a pre-treatment, increasing the skin's tolerance to sunburn. In fact, one gram of omega-3 fatty acids daily may reduce the risk of getting burned by the sun's ultraviolet rays.

OMEGA-3 FROM THE INSIDE OUT

Omega-3 fatty acids act on the body's cellular structure, enabling the benefits to push their way to the surface where they can do the most external good.

The consensus is that omega-3 is incorporated into cell membranes, making them more fluid. Every cell membrane has a layer of fat surrounding it. Receptors stick out of the cell, essentially floating in that membrane of fat. If the cell membrane is covered in bad fat, then the receptors become inflexible and don't deliver what the body needs. Omega-3, an essential fatty acid that comes only from good food, works to allow receptors to function more smoothly, thus delivering the right messages to the brain and to the body in general. If the cells of the skin are told that they're hydrated and lush, then the skin responds accordingly, as do the finger and toenails, as well as the hair.

A diet rich in essential fatty acids will help encourage beauty from the inside out through internal hydration. Think of it this way: The body is like the planet. On the outside of the planet there is 75 percent water, while the layer of the planet just beneath the surface can hold up to 100 percent of the moisture it absorbs, dispensing it as necessary to feed the plants, animals and humans above. The skin is much the same. Our bodies are as much as 60 percent water. While the surface of the skin itself is waterproof, its truest source of moisture comes from within the body. This is why we drink fluids, and why we can't live for more than 8 to 10 days without hydration. In fact, nothing can live without water. Water makes the hills green, the flowers bloom, and the earth smile. It makes skin supple and hair healthier.

It's amazing to also know that external beauty suffers when there is a lack of essential fatty acids within the body.

Proper nutrients are what allow the body to thrive, both internally and externally. A healthy body can mean healthy skin, nails and hair. After all, the first thing we notice about each other is our outward appearance. No one ever says: "Hey, nice pancreas," or "What a beautiful vascular structure you have." Rather, we hear: "Your skin is like porcelain," or "Your hair is so shiny and healthy looking," or "Did you just get your nails done?" and "What have you done to look so good?"

Imagine being able to respond by saying "I owe it all to 100 percent fish oil."

OMEGA-3: COMING SOON TO A CREAM NEAR YOU

If omega-3s can create such an abundantly rich environment inside the body, one that enables the body to help heal itself, wouldn't it be amazing if such a process was available as a topical treatment? The possibility exists and dermatologists and research scientists are working on such a cream as this goes to print.

Imagine the possibilities of having internal essential fatty acids working together with external omega-3s. If skin can become more supple, nails can become strong, and hair can achieve health and vibrancy because of an increase in omega-3 inside, imagine what it will do when smoothed on the skin.

Beauty is waiting.

THE BEAUTY OF OMEGA-3

Over 2,000 studies have demonstrated the wide range of potential health issues associated with omega-3 deficiencies—diabetes, cancer, arthritis, inflammatory diseases, depression, heart disease, hypertension, memory problems, weight gain, some allergies and now even skin conditions. Researchers believe that nearly 60 percent of American adults are deficient in omega-3 fatty acids, and that 20 percent have so little present in their bloodstreams that tests cannot detect it. The human brain, which is more than 60 percent fat, is rich in good kinds of fat like that received from omega-3 fatty acids. When the body, and consequently the brain, is deprived of these essential fatty acids, it suffers. The brain may not seem as sharp, and the body may show signs of eczema, thick patches of skin, cracked heels and even dandruff.

The external issues associated with omega-3 deficiency include skin problems that range from dryness to the dreaded alligator skin or pimply chicken skin on the back of the arms. Face it. Skin that looks like the floor of a desert that has seen no rain for years tends to be scarred, cracked, and unattractive. Cracked skin on heels or fingertips mean that it's not getting enough hydration, and all the moisturizing creams and lotions in the world will do next to nothing to help. These types of topical solutions provide temporary relief to be sure, but do not address the primary cause of the problem, namely omega-3 depletion.

Other problems include soft nails or brittle nails that split easily, a dry scalp that flakes in dandruff, and dull, thinning hair.

The solution may found in fat, fish and oil, three words not normally associated with beauty. These terms may actually send shivers through that 60-percent-fat brain, but ingesting enough foods or supplements to increase levels of omega-3 can be a beautiful thing. Therein lies the true beauty of this miraculous essential fatty acid.

References

Part I
Chapter 1

1 Henzen, C. "Fish oil--healing principle in the Eskimo diet?" *Schweiz Rundsch Med Prax,* 1995;84(1):11-15.

2 Chen L.Y., et al. "Effect of stable fish oil on arterial thrombogenesis, platelet aggregation, and superoxide dismutase activity." *J Cardiovasc Pharmacol,* Mar 2000;35(3):502-505.

2 Yosefy, C., et al. "The effect of fish oil on hypertension, plasma lipids and hemostasis in hypertensive, obese, dyslipidemic patients with and without diabetes mellitus." *Prostaglandins Leukot Essent Fatty Acids,* Aug 1999;61(2):83-87.

3 McCarty, M.F. "Fish oil may be an antidote for the cardiovascular risk of smoking." *Med Hypotheses,* Apr 1996;46(4):337-347.

4 Harris, W.S. "Dietary fish oil and blood lipids." *Curr Opin Lipidol,* Feb 1996;7(1):3-7.

5 Cen, X., & Wang, R. "Study on the dose-effect relationship of hypolipidemic effect of deep sea fish oil." *Wei Sheng Yen Chiu* Sept 1997; 26(5):337-339.

6 Siscovick, D.S., et al. "Dietary intake of long-chain n-3 polyunsaturated fatty acids and the risk of primary cardiac arrest." *Am J Clin Nutr,* Jan 2000;71:208S-212S.

8 Nasa, Y., et al. "Long-term supplementation with eicosapentaenoic acid salvages cardiomyocytes from hypoxia/reoxygenation-induced injury in rats fed with fish-oil-deprived diet." *Jpn J Pharmacol* June 1998;77(2):137-146.

9 Singh, R.B., et al. "Randomized, double-blind, placebo-controlled trial of fish oil and mustard oil in patients with suspected acute myocardial infarction: the Indian experiment of infarct survival–4." *Cardiovasc Drugs Ther,* July 1997; 11(3):485-491.

10 Sellmayer, A., et al. "Effects of dietary fish oil on ventricular premature complexes." *Am J Cardiol,* Nov 1995;76(12):974-977.

11 McCarty, M.F. "Vascular nitric oxide, sex hormone replacement, and fish oil may help to prevent Alzheimer's disease by suppressing synthesis of acute-phase cytokines." *Med Hypotheses,* Nov 1999;53(5):369-374.

12 Olsen, S.F., et al. "Randomised clinical trials of fish oil supplementation in high risk pregnancies–Fish Oil Trials In Pregnancy (FOTIP) Team." *BJOG,* Mar 2000;107(3):382-395.

13 Jeyarajah, D.R., et al. "Docosahexaenoic acid, a component of fish oil, inhibits nitric oxide production in vitro." *J Surg Res,* May 1999;83(2): 147-150.

14 Fortin, P.R., et al. "Validation of a metanalysis: the effects of fish oil in rheumatoid arthritis." *J Clin Epidemiol,* Nov 1995;48(11):1379-1390.

15 Kremer, J.M., et al. "Effects of high-dose fish oil on rheumatoid arthritis after stopping nonsteroidal anti-inflammatory drugs." Clinical and immune correlates. *Arthritis Rheum,* Aug 1995;38(8):1107-1114.

16 Lau, C.S., et al. "Effects of fish oil supplementation on non-steroidal anti-inflammatory drug requirement in patients with mild rheumatoid arthritis–a double-blind placebo controlled study." *Br J Rheumatol,* Nov 1993; 32(11):982-989.

17 Frati, C., et al. "Association of etretinate and fish oil in psoriasis therapy. Inhibition of hypertriglyceridemia resulting from retinoid therapy after fish oil supplementation." *Acta Derm Venereol Suppl* (Stockh), 1994;186:151-153.

18 Caygill, C.P., et al. "Fat, fish, fish oil and cancer." *Br J Cancer,* July 1996;74(1):159-164.

19 Kenler, A.S., et al. "Early enteral feeding in postsurgical cancer patients. Fish oil structured lipid-based polymeric formula versus a standard polymeric formula." *Ann Surg,* March 1996;223(3):316-333.

20 "Fish-oil supplementation reduces intestinal hyperproliferation in persons at risk for colon cancer." *Nutr Rev,* Aug 1993;51(8):241-243

21 Burns, C.P., et al. "Phase I clinical study of fish oil fatty acid capsules for patients with cancer cachexia: cancer and leukemia group B study 9473." *Clin Cancer Res*, Dec 1999;5(12):3942-3947.

22 Friedberg, C.E., et al. "Fish oil and glycemic control in diabetes. A metanalysis." *Diabetes Care*, Apr 1998;21(4):494-500.

23 Sirtori, C.R., et al. "N-3 fatty acids do not lead to an increased diabetic risk in patients with hyperlipidemia and abnormal glucose tolerance. Italian Fish Oil Multicenter Study." *Am J Clin Nutr*, Jun 1997;65(6):1874-1881.

24 Donadio, J.V. Jr. "Use of fish oil to treat patients with immunoglobulin and nephropathy." *Am J Clin Nutr*, Jan 2000;71(1 Suppl): 373S-375S.

25 Drago, L. "Effects of three different fish oil formulations on Helicobacter pylori growth and viability: in vitro study." *J Chemother*, Jun 1999;11(3):207-210.

26 Chen, D. & Auborn, K. "Fish oil constituent docosa-hexa-enoic acid selectively inhibits growth of human papillomavirus immortalized keratinocytes." *Carcinogenesis*, Feb 1999;20(2):249-254.

27 McCarty, M.F., "Magnesium taurate and fish oil for prevention of migraine." *Med Hypotheses*, Dec 1996;47(6):461-466.

28 Gibson, R.A. "The effect of diets containing fish and fish oils on disease risk factors in humans." *Aust N Z J Med*, Aug 1988;18(5):713-722.

29 Levine, Barbara S. "Most frequently asked questions about DHA." *Nutrition Today*, Nov/Dec 1997;32: 248-249.

30 Taioli, E., et al. "Dietary habits and breast cancer: a comparative study of the United States and Italian data." *Nutrition and Cancer*, 1991;16:259-265.

31 Yanagi, S., et al. "Sodium butyrate inhibits the enhancing effect of high fat on mammary tumorigenesis." *Oncology*, 1993;50(4):201-204.

32 Yam, D., et al. "Diet and disease--the Israeli paradox: possible dangers of a high omega-6 polyunsaturated fatty acid diet." *Israeli J Med Sci.*1996;32:1134-1143.

Chapter 2

34 Okuyama, H., et al. "Dietary fatty acids - the N-6 / N-3 balance and chronic elderly diseases. Excess linoleic acid and relative N-3 deficiency syndrome seen in Japan." *Prog Lipid Res*, 1997;3(4):409-457.

Part II
Chapter 1

35 Simon, J. A., et al. "Serum fatty acids and the risk of coronary heart disease."American *Journal of Epidemiology*, Sept 1995;142(5):469-476.

36 De Caterina, R., et al. "Antiarrhythmic effects of omega-3 fatty acids: from epidemiology to bedside." *American Heart Journal*, Sept 2003; 164:420-430.

37 Marchioli, R., et al. "Early protection against sudden death by n-3 polyunsaturated fatty acids after myocardial infarction: time-course analysis of the results of the Gruppo Italiano per lo Studio della Sopravvivenza nell'Infarto Miocardico (GISSI)-Prevenzione." *Circulation*, 2002;105(16):1897-1903.

38 Albert, C.M., Campos, H., et al. "Blood levels of long-chain n-3 fatty acids and the risk of sudden death." *N Engl J Med*, 2002;346(15): 1113-1118.

39 Simopoulos, A. "Omega-3 fatty acids in health and disease and in growth and development." *American Journal of Clinical Nutrition*, 1991;54:438-463.

40 Pepping, J. "Omega-3: essential fatty acids." *American Journal of Health-System Pharmacy*, Vol. 56, Apr 1999;56: 719-724.

41 Uauy-Dagach, R. & Valenzuela, A. "Marine oils: the health benefits of n-3 fatty acids." *Nutrition Reviews*, Vol. 54, November 1996, pp. S102-S108.

42 Connor, W. E. "Importance of n-3 fatty acids in health and disease." American Journal of Clinical Nutrition, Jan 2000;171:171S-175S.

43 Daviglus, M. L., et al. "Fish consumption and the 30-year risk of fatal myocardial infarction." *New England Journal of Medicine*, Apr 1997;336:1046-1053.

44 Christensen, J. H., et al. "Effect of fish oil on heart rate variability in survivors of myocardial infarction." *British Medical Journal*, March 1996;312:677-678.

45 Simon, J. A., et al. "Serum fatty acids and the risk of coronary heart disease." American *Journal of Epidemiology*, Sept 1995;142(5):469-476.

46 Flaten, H., et al. "Fish-oil concentrate: effects of variables related to cardiovascular disease." *American Journal of Clinical Nutrition*, 1990;52:300-306.

47 Christensen, J. H., et al. "Heart rate variability and fatty acid content of blood cell membranes: a dose-response study with n-3 fatty acids." *American Journal of Clinical Nutrition*, Sept 1999;70:331-337.

48 "Dietary supplementation with n-3 polyunsaturated fatty acids and vitamin E after myocardial infarction: results of the GISSI-Prevenzion trial." *The Lancet*, Aug 1999;354: 447-455.

49 Brown, M. "Do vitamin E and fish oil protect against ischaemic heart disease?" *The Lancet*, Aug 1999;354:441-442.

50 von Schacky, C., et al. "The effect of dietary omega-3 fatty acids on coronary atherosclerosis." *Annals of Internal Medicine*, Apr. 1999;130:554-562.

51 Albert, C. M., et al. "Fish consumption and risk of sudden cardiac death." Journal of the *American Medical Association*, Jan 1998;279:23-28.

52 Kromhout, D. "Fish consumption and sudden cardiac death." *Journal of the American Medical Association*, Jan 1998;297:65-66.

53 Siscovick, D. S., et al. "Dietary intake and cell membrane levels of long-chain n-3 polyunsaturated fatty acids and the risk of primary cardiac arrest." *Journal of the American Medical Association*, 1995;274(17):1363-1367.

54 Appel, L. J., et al. "Does supplementation of diet with 'fish oil' reduce blood pressure?" *Archives of Internal Medicine*, 1993;153:1429-1438.

55 Appel, L.J., Moore, T.J., et al. "A clinical trial of the effects of dietary patterns on blood pressure." *N Engl J Med*, 1997;336:1117–1124.

56 Svetkey, L.P., Simons-Morton, D., et al. "Effects of dietary patterns on blood pressure: a subgroup analysis of the Dietary Approaches to Stop Hypertension (DASH) randomized clinical trial." *Arch Intern Med*, 1999;159:285–93.

57 Jee, S.H., He, J., et al. "The effect of chronic coffee drinking on blood pressure. A metanalysis of controlled clinical trials." *Hypertension*, 1999;33:647–652.

58 Keil, U., Liese, A., et al. "Alcohol, blood pressure and hypertension." *Novartis Round Symp*, 1998;216:125–144.

59 Young, D.R., Appel, L.G, et al. "The effect of aerobic exercise and T'ai Chi on blood pressure in older people: results of a randomized trial." *J Am Geriatr Soc*, 1999;47:277–284.

60 Griffith, L.E., Guyatt, G.H., et al. "The influence of dietary and nondietary calcium supplementation on blood pressure. An updated metanalysis of randomized controlled trials." *Am J Hypertens*, 1999;12:84–92.

61 Resnick, L.M. "The role of dietary calcium in hypertension: a hierarchical review." *Am J Hypertens*, 1999;12:99-112.

62 Motoyama, T., Sano, H., et al. "Oral magnesium supplementation in patients with essential hypertension." *Hypertension*, 1989;13:227–232.

63 Patki, P.S., Singh, J., et al. "Efficacy of potassium and magnesium in essential hypertension: a double-blind, placebo controlled, crossover study." *BMJ*, 1990;301:521–523.

64 Digiesi, V., Cantini, F.,et al. "Mechanism of action of coenzyme Q_{10} in essential hypertension." *Curr Ther Res*, 1992;51:668–672.

65 Folkers, K., Drzewoski, J., et al. "Bioenergetics in clinical medicine. XVI. Reduction of hypertension in patients by therapy with coenzyme Q_{10}." *Res Commun Chem Pathol Pharmacol*, 1981;31:129–140.

66 Langsjoen, P., Willis, R., et al. "Treatment of essential hypertension with coenzyme Q_{10}." *Mol Aspects Med*, 1994;15(Suppl):S265–S272.

67 Digiesi, V., Cantini, F., et al. "Coenzyme Q_{10} in essential hypertension." *Molec Aspects Med*, 1994;15(Suppl):S257–S263.

68 Digiesi, V., Cantini, F., et al. "Effect of coenzyme Q_{10} on essential arterial hypertension." *Curr Ther Res*, 1990;47:841–845.

69 Singh, R.B., Niaz, M.A., et al. "Effect of hydrosoluble coenzyme Q_{10} on blood pressures and insulin resistance in hypertensive patients with coronary artery disease." *J Hum Hypertens*, 1999;13:203–208.

70 Morris, M.C., Sacks, F., et al. "Does fish oil lower blood pressure? A metanalysis of controlled trials." *Circulation*, 1993;88:523–533. 71 Prichard, B.N., Smith, C.C.T., et al. "Fish oils and cardiovascular disease." *BMJ*, 1995; 310: 819–820.

71 Prichard, B.N., Smith, C.C.T., el at. "Fish oils and cardiovascular disease." BMJ, 1995:310: 819-820.

72 von Schacky, C., Fischer, S., et al. "Long-term effects of dietary marine omega-3 fatty acids upon plasma and cellular lipids, platelet function, and eicosanoid formation in humans." *J Clin Invest*, 1985;76:1626–1631.

73 Leaf, A. & Weber, P.C. "Cardiovascular effects of n-3 fatty acids." *N Engl J Med*, 1988;318:549–557.

74 Adler, A.J. & Holub, B.J. "Effect of garlic and fish-oil supplementation on serum lipid and lipoprotein concentrations in hypercholesterolemic men." *Am J Clin Nutr*, 1997;65:445–450.

75 Haglund, O., Luostarinen, R., et al. "The effects of fish oil on triglycerides, cholesterol, fibrinogen and malondialdehyde in humans supplemented with vitamin E." *J Nutr*, 1991; 121:165–169.

76 Oostenbrug, G.S., Mensink, R.P., et al. "A moderate in vivo vitamin E supplement counteracts the fish-oil induced increase in in-vitro oxidation of human low-density lipoproteins." *Am J Clin Nutr*, 1993;57:827S.

77 He, K., Rimm, E. B., et al. "Fish consumption and risk of stroke in men." *Journal of the American Medical Association*, 2002;288:3130-3136.

78 The study adds to a growing body of research into the effect of fish on stroke risk for men and women. One recent report found that women who ate at least five servings of fish a week had a 62 percent lower risk of stroke, compared with those who ate fish less than once a month.

79 Saynor, R., Verel, D., et al. "The long-term effect of dietary supplementation with fish lipid concentrate on serum lipids, bleeding time, platelets and angina." *Atherosclerosis*, 1984;50:3–10.

80 Mehta, J.L., Lopez, L.M., et al. "Dietary supplementation with omega-3 polyunsaturated fatty acids in patients with stable coronary heart disease. Effects on indices of platelet and neutrophil function and exercise performance." *Am J Med*, 1988;84:45–52.

81 Wander, R.C., Du, S.H., et al. "Alpha-tocopherol influences in vivo indices of lipid peroxidation in postmenopausal women given fish oil." *J Nutr*, 1996;126:643–652.

82 Oostenbrug, G.S., Mensink, R.P., et al. "A moderate in vivo vitamin E supplement counteracts the fish-oil-induced increase in in vitro oxidation of human low-density lipoproteins." *Am J Clin Nutr*, 1993;57:827S.

Chapter 2

83 Cave, W.T. Jr. "Omega-3 polyunsaturated fatty acids in rodent models of breast cancer." *Breast Cancer Res Treat* 1997;46(2-3):239-246.

84 Bagga, D., Anders, K.H., et al. "Long-chain n-3-to-n-6 polyunsaturated fatty acid ratios in breast adipose tissue from women with and without breast cancer." *Nutr Cancer* 2002;42(2):180-185.

85 Maillard, V., Bougnoux, P., et al. "N-3 and N-6 fatty acids in breast adipose tissue and relative risk of breast cancer in a case-control study in Tours, France." *Int J Cancer,* 2002;98(1):78-83.

86 Fernandez-Banares, F., Esteve, M., et al. "Changes of the mucosal n-3 and n-6 fatty acid status occur early in the colorectal adenoma-carcinoma sequence." *Gut* 1996;38(2):254-259.

87 Anti, M., Armelao, F., et al. "Effects of different doses of fish oil on rectal cell proliferation in patients with sporadic colonic adenomas." *Gastroenterology,* 1994;107(6):1709-1718.

88 Karmali, R.A. "Historical perspective and potential use of n-3 fatty acids in therapy of cancer cachexia." *Nutrition,* 1996;12(1 Suppl):S2-4.

89 Stoll, B.A. "N-3 fatty acids and lipid peroxidation in breast cancer inhibition." *Br J Nutr,* 2002;87(3):193-198.

90 Rose, D.P. & Connolly, J.M. "Omega-3 fatty acids as cancer chemopreventive agents." *Pharmacol Ther,* 1999;83(3):217-244.

91 Hardman, W.E. "Omega-3 fatty acids to augment cancer therapy." *J Nutr,* 2002;132(11 Suppl):3508S-3512S.

92 Takezaki, T., et al. "Dietary factors and lung cancer risk in Japanese with special reference to fish consumption and adenocarcinomas." *British Journal of Cancer,* 2001;84(9):1199- 1206.

93 Ibid.

94 Kobayashi, M., Sasaki, S., et al. "Serum n-3 fatty acids, fish consumption and cancer mortality in six Japanese populations in Japan and Brazil." *Jpn J Cancer Res,* 1999;90(9):914-921.

95 Terry, P., Rohan, T.E., et al. "Fish consumption and breast cancer risk." *Nutr Cancer,* 2002;44(1):1-6.

96 Holmes, M.D., Colditz, G.A., et al. "Meat, fish and egg intake and risk of breast cancer." *Int J Cancer,* 2003;104(2):221-227.

97 Stripp, C., Overvad, K., et al. "Fish intake is positively associated with breast cancer incidence rate." *J Nutr,* 2003;133(11):3664-3669.

98 Caygill, C.P., Charlett, A., et al. "Fat, fish, fish oil and cancer." *Br J Cancer,* 1996;74(1):159-164.

99 Tavani, A., Pelucchi, C., et al. "N-3 polyunsaturated fatty acid intake and cancer risk in Italy and Switzerland." *Int J Cancer,* 2003;105(1):113-116.

100 Caygill, C.P. & Hill, M.J. "Fish, n-3 fatty acids and human colorectal and breast cancer mortality." *Eur J Cancer Prev,* 1995;4(4):329-332.

101 Yang, C.X., Takezaki, T., et al. "Fish consumption and colorectal cancer: a case-reference study in Japan." *Eur J Cancer Prev,* 2003;12(2): 109-115.

102 Bougnoux, P., et al. "Alpha-linolenic acid content of adipose breast tissue: a host determinant of the risk of early metastasis in breast cancer." *Br J Cancer.* 1994; 70: 330-334.

103 Goodstine, S.L., Zheng, T., et al. "Dietary (n-3)/(n-6) fatty acid ratio: possible relationship to premenopausal but not postmenopausal breast cancer risk in U.S. women." *J Nut.* May 2003;133(5):1409-1414.

104 Bougnoux, P., et al. "Alpha-linolenic acid content of adipose breast tissue: a host determinant of the risk of early metastasis in breast cancer." *Br J Cancer,* 1994; 70:330-334.

105 Augustsson, K., Michaud, D.S., et al. "A prospective study of intake of fish and marine fatty acids and prostate cancer." *Cancer Epidemiol Biomarkers Pre,.* Jan 2003;12(1):64-67.

106 Kolonel, L.N., et al. "Dietary fat and prostate cancer: current status." *J Natl Cancer Inst,* 1999;91(5):414-428.

107 Harvei, S., et al. "Prediagnostic level of fatty acids in serum phospholipids: omega-3 and omega-6 fatty acids and the risk of prostate cancer." *Int J Cancer,* 1997;71(4):545-551.

108 Godley, P.A., et al. "Biomarkers of essential fatty acid consumption and risk of prostatic carcinoma." *Cancer Epidemiol Biomarkers Prev,* 1996;5(11):889-895.

109 Giovannucci, E., et al. "A prospective study of dietary fat and risk of prostate cancer." *J Natl Cancer Inst,* 1993 ;85(19):1571-1579.

110 Gann, P.H., et al. "Prospective study of plasma fatty acids and risk of prostate cancer." *J Natl Cancer Inst,* 1994;86(4):281-286.

111 Andersson, S.O., et al. "Energy, nutrient intake and prostate cancer risk: a population-based case-control study in Sweden." *Int J Cancer,* 1996;68(6):716-722.

112 Takezaki, T., Inoue, M., et al. "Diet and lung cancer risk from a 14-year population-based prospective study in Japan: with special reference to fish consumption." *Nutr Cancer,* 2003;45(2):160-167.

113 Falconer, J.S., et al. "Effect of eicosapentaenoic acid and other fatty acids on the growth in vitro of human pancreatic cancer cell lines." *Br J Cancer,* 1994;69:826-832.

114 Bougnoux, P. "N-3 polyunsaturated fatty acids and cancer." *Curr Opin Clin Nutr Metab Care,* Mar 1999;2(2):121-126.

115 Schauss, A. "Fish oils." *Textbook of Natural Medicine,* Pizzorno, J., and Murray, M., eds. London: Churchill Livingstone, 1999, p. 773.

116 Barber, M.D., Ross, J.A., et al. "The effect of an oral nutritional supplement enriched with fish oil on weight-loss in patients with pancreatic cancer." *Br J Cancer,* Sept 1999;81(1):80-86.

117 Gogos, C.A., Ginopoulos, P., et al. "Dietary omega-3 polyunsaturated fatty acids plus vitamin E restore immunodeficiency and prolong survival for severely ill patients with generalized malignancy: a randomized control trial." *Cancer* Jan 1998;82(2):395-402.

Chapter 3

118 Simopolous, A. *The Omega Plan.* New York: HarperCollins, 1998, 86-98.

119 Simopolous, A., et al. "Essential fatty acids predict metabolites of serotonin and dopamine in CSF among healthy controls, early and late onset alcoholics." *Biol Psychiatry,* 1998;44:235-242.

120 Hibbeln, J.R., et al. "A replication study of violent and non-violent subjects: CSF metabolites of serotonin and dopamine are predicted by plasma essential fatty acids." *Biol Psychiatry,* 1998; 44: 243-249.

121 Bruinsma, K.A. & Taren, D. L. "Dieting, essential fatty acid intake, and depression." *Nutrition Reviews,* Vol. 58, 2000;58:98-108.

122 Stillwell, W. & Wassall, S.R. "Docosahexaenoic acid: membrane properties of a unique fatty acid." *Chem Phys Lipids,* 2003;126(1):1-27.

123 Colin, A., Reggers, J., et al. "Lipids, depression and suicide." *Encephale,* 2003;29(1):49-58.

124 Hibbeln, J.R. "Fish consumption and major depression." *Lancet,* 1998;351:1213.

125 Mischoulon, D. & Fava, M. "Docosahexanoic acid and omega-3 fatty acids in depression." *Psychiatr Clin North Am,* 2000;23(4):785-794.

126 Mes, M., et al. "Fatty acid composition in major depression: Decreased omega-3 fractions in cholesteryl esters and increased C20:4 omega-6/C20:5 omega-3 ratio in cholesteryl esters and phospholipids." *J Affect Disord,* 1996;38:35-46.

127 Adams, P.B., et al. "Arachadonic acid to eicosapentaneoic acid ratio in blood correlates positively with clinical symptoms of depression." *Lipids,* 1996;31:S157-S161.

128 Edwards, R., et al. "Omega-3 polyunsaturated fatty acids in the diet and in the red blood cell membranes of depressed patients." *J Affect Disord,* 1998;48:149-155.

129 Mamalakis, G., Tornaritis, M., et al. "Depression and adipose essential polyunsaturated fatty acids." *Prostaglandins Leukot Essent Fatty Acids,* 2002;67(5):311-318.

130 Holman, R.T., et al. "Deficiency of essential fatty acids and membrane fluidity during pregnancy and lactation." *Proc Natl Acad Sci,* 1991;88:4835-4839.

131 Ibid.

132 Virkkunen, M.E., et al. "Plasma phospholipid essential fatty acids and prostaglandins in alcoholic, habitually violent, and impulsive offenders." *Biological Psychiatry,* 1987;22:1087-1096.

133 Kaplan, J.R., et al. "The effects of fat and cholesterol on social behavior in monkeys." *Psychosomatic Medicine,* 1991;53:634-642.

134 Hamazaki, T.S., et al. "The effect of docosahexaenoic acid on aggression in young adults." *J of Clinical Investigation,* 1996;97(4):1129-1134.

135 Hibbeln, J.R., et al. "A replication study of violent and non-violent subjects: CSF metabolites of serotonin and dopamine are predicted by plasma essential fatty acids." *Biol Psychiatry,* 1998;44:243-249.

136 Hamazak, T., Thienprasert, A., et al. "The effect of docosahexaenoic acid on aggression in elderly Thai subjects—a placebo-controlled double-blind study." *Nutr Neurosci,* 2002;5(1):37-41.

137 Gesch, C.B., Hammond, S.M., et al. "Influence of supplementary vitamins, minerals and essential fatty acids on the antisocial behaviour of young adult prisoners. Randomised, placebo-controlled trial." *Br J Psychiatry,* 2002;181:22-28.

138 Stoll, A.L., Severus, W.E., et al. "Omega 3 fatty acids in bipolar disorder: a preliminary double-blind, placebo-controlled trial." *Arch Gen Psychiatry,* 1999;56(5):407-412.

139 Noaghiul, S. & Hibbeln, J.R. "Cross-national comparisons of seafood consumption and rates of bipolar disorders." *Am J Psychiatry,* 2003;160(12):2222-2227.

140 Hoffer, A. & Osmond, H. "Chronic schizophrenic patients treated ten years or more." *Journal of Orthomolecular Medicine,* 1993; 8:7-37.

141 Corrigan, F.M., Van Rhijn, A., et al. "Essential fatty acids in Alzheimer's disease." *Ann N Y Acad Sci,* 1991;640:250-252.

142 Klein W.L., et al. "Targeting small Aß oligomers: the solution to an Alzheimer's disease conundrum?" *Trends Neurosci,* 2001;24:219-224.

143 McCarty, M.F. "Vascular nitric oxide, sex hormone replacement, and fish oil may help to prevent Alzheimer's disease by suppressing synthesis of acute-phase cytokines." *Med Hypotheses,* 1999;53(5):369-374.

Chapter 4

144 Long, M. & Barrett, P. "Lawsuit is filed against Novartis on Ritalin sales." *The Wall Street Journal Europe,* May 15, 2000: 4.

145 Adesman, A. "Does my child need Ritalin?" *Newsweek,* April 24, 2000:81.

146 Parker-Pope, T "Drug firms research kids' one-a-day Ritalin." *The Wall Street Journal Europe,* May 15, 2000: 31.

147 Mitchell, E.A., Aman, M.G., et al. "Clinical characteristics and serum essential fatty acid levels in hyperactive children." *Clin Pediatr* (Phila), 1987;26(8):406-411.

148 Pelsser, L.M. & Buitelaar, J.K. "Favourable effect of a standard elimination diet on the behavior of young children with attention deficit hyperactivity disorder (ADHD): a pilot study." *Ned Tijdschr Geneeskd,* 2002;146(52): 2543-2547.

149 Breakey, J. "The role of diet and behaviour in childhood." *J Paediatr Child Health,* 1997; 33(3):190-194.

150 Rudin, D. & Felix, C. *Omega-3 Oils: A Practical Guide.* Garden City Park, NY: Avery Publishing, 1996.

151 Colquhoun, I. & Bunday, S. "A lack of essential fatty acids as a possible cause of hyperactivity in children." *Med Hypotheses,* 1981;7(5):673-679.

152 Stevens, L.J., Zentall, S.S., et al. "Essential fatty acid metabolism in boys with attention-deficit hyperactivity disorder." *Am J Clin Nutr,* 1995;62(4):761-768.

153 Burgess, J.R., Stevens, L., et al. "Long-chain polyunsaturated fatty acids in children with attention-deficit hyperactivity disorder." *Am J Clin Nutr,* 2000;71(1 Suppl):327S-30S.

154 Neuringer, M. & Conner, W.E. "N-3 fatty acids in the brain and retina: evidence for their essentiality." *Nutrition Reviews,* 1985;44:285-294.

155 Tinoco, J. "Dietary requirement and function of alpha-linolenic acid in animals." *Prog Lipid Res,* 1982;21:1-45.

156 Enslen, M., et al. "Effect of low intake of n-3 fatty acids during the development of brain phospholipid fatty acid composition and exploratory behavior in rats." *Lipids,* 1991;26:203-208.

157 Reisbick, S., et al. "Home cage behavior or rhesus monkeys with long-term deficiency of omega-3 fatty acids." *Physiol Behav,* 1994;55:231-239.

158 Colquhoun, I. & Bunday, S. "A lack of essential fatty acids as a possible cause of hyperactivity in children." *Med Hypotheses,* 1981;7:673-679.

159 Mitchell E.A., et al. "Essential fatty acids and maladjusted behaviour in children." *Prostaglandins Leukot Med,* 1983;12(3):281-287.

160 Mitchell E.A., et al. "Clinical characteristics and serum essential fatty acid levels in hyperactive children." *Clin Pediatr,* 1987;26:406-411.

161 Stevens, L.J., Zentall, S.S., et al. "Essential fatty acid metabolism in boys with attention-deficit hyperactivity disorder." *American Journal of Clinical Nutrition,* 1995;62:761-768.

162 Stevens, L.J., Zentall, S.S., et al. "Omega-3 fatty acids in boys with behavior, learning, and health problems." *Physiology & Behavior,* 1996;59(4-5):915-920.

163 Bekaröglu, M., et al. "Relationships between serum free fatty acids and zinc, and attention deficit hyperactivity disorder: a research note." *J Child Psychol Psychiatry,* 1996;37(2):225-227.

164 *Developmental Medicine & Child Neurology,* 2000;42:174-181.

165 Stordy, B. J. "Dark adaptation, motor skills, docosahexaenoic acid, and dyslexia." *American Journal of Clinical Nutrition,* 2000;71:323S-326S.

Chapter 5

166 Olsen, S.F. & Secher, N.J. "Low consumption of seafood in early pregnancy as a risk factor for preterm delivery: prospective cohort study." *British Medical Journal,* 2002;324:1-5.

167 Fidler, N., et al. "Docosahexaenoic acid transfer into human milk after dietary supplementation: a randomized clinical trial." *Journal of Lipid Research,* 2000;41:1376-1383.

168 Makrides, M. & Gibson, R.A. "Long-chain polyunsaturated fatty acid requirements during pregnancy and lactation." *American Journal of Clinical Nutrition,* 2000;71: 307S-311S.

169 Cunnane, Stephen C., et al. "Breast-fed infants achieve a higher rate of brain and whole body docosahexaenoate accumulation than formula-fed infants not consuming dietary docosahexaenoate." *Lipids,* 2000;35:105-111.

170 Jensen, Craig L., et al. "Effect of docosahexaenoic acid supplementation of lactating women on the fatty acid composition of breast milk lipids and maternal and infant plasma phospholipids." *American Journal of Clinical Nutrition,* 2000;71:292S-299S.

171 Carlson, S.E. "Long-chain polyunsaturated fatty acids and development of human infants." *Acta Paediatr Suppl,* 1999;430:72-73.

172 Levine, B.S. Most frequently asked questions about DHA. *Nutrition Today,* 1997;32:248-249.

173 Connor, W.E., et al. "Increased docosahexaenoic acid levels in human newborn infants by administration of sardines and fish oil during pregnancy." *Lipids,* 1996;3: S183-S187.

174 Agostoni, C., et al. "Docosahexaenoic acid status and developmental quotient of healthy term infants." *Lancet,* 1995;346:638.

Chapter 6

175 Burkitt, D. & Trowell, H. *Western Diseases: Their Emergence and Prevention.* Cambridge: Harvard University Press, 1981.

176 Vessby, B., et al. "The risk to develop NIDDM is related to the fatty acid composition of the serum cholesterol esters." *Diabetes,* 1994; 43(11):1353-1357.

177 Hainault, I.M., et al. "Fish oil in a high lard diet prevents obesity, hyperlipidemia, and adipocyte insulin resistance in rats." *Annals of New York Academy of Sciences,* year;1993;683: 98-101.

178 Ikemoto, S., et al. "High-fat diet-induced hyperglycemia and obesity in mice: Differential effects of dietary oils." *Metabolism,* 1996; 45(12):1539-1546.

179 Ibid.

180 Sirtori, C.R. & Galli, C. "N-3 fatty acids and diabetes." *Biomed Pharmacother,* 2002;56(8):397-406

181 Coste,T.C., Gerbi, A., et al. "Neuroprotective effect of docosahexaenoic acid-enriched phospholipids in experimental diabetic neuropathy." *Diabetes,* 2003;52(10):2578-2585.

182 Storlien, L.H. "Skeletal muscle membrane lipids and insulin resistance." *Lipids* 1996;31: S-261-265.

183 Torjesen, P.A., et al. "Lifestyle changes may reverse development of the insulin resistance syndrome." Diabetes Care, 1997;30:26-31.

184 Fanaian, M., et al. "The effect of modified fat diet on insulin resistance and metabolic parameter sin type II diabetes." *Diabetologia,* 1996;39(1):A7.

Chapter 7

185 Deutch, B. "Menstrual pain in Danish women

correlated with low n-3 polyunsaturated fatty acid intake." *Eur J Clin Nutr,* 1995;49(7):508-516.

186 Kruger M.C., Coetzer, H., et al. "Calcium, gamma-linolenic acid and eicosapentaenoic acid supplementation in senile osteoporosis." *Aging,* 1998;10:385–394.

187 Galeao, R. "La dysmenorrhee, syndrome multiforme." *Gynecologie,* 1974;25:125 [in French].

188 Harel, Z., Biro F.M., et al. "Supplementation with omega-3 polyunsaturated fatty acids in the management of dysmenorrhea in adolescents." *Am J Obstet Gynecol,* 1996;174:1335–1338.

189 Murray, M. & Pizzorno, J. *Encyclopedia of Natural Medicine.* Rocklin: Prima Publishing, 1998, 448-454, 763-769.

190 Ziboh, V.A. "Implications of dietary oils and polyunsaturated fatty acids in the management of cutaneous disorders." *Arch Dermatol,* 1989;125(2):241-245.

191 Veien, N.K., Hattel, T., et al. "Dermatoses in coffee drinkers." *Cutis* 1987;40:421–422.

192 Bjørneboe, A., Søyland, E., et al. "Effect of dietary supplementation with eicosapentaenoic acid in the treatment of atopic dermatitis." *Br J Dermatol,* 1987;117:463–469.

193 Bjørneboe, A., Søyland, E., et al. "Effect of n-3 fatty acid supplement to patients with atopic dermatitis." *J Intern Med Suppl,* 1989;225:233–236.

194 Søyland, E., Rajka, G., et al. "The effect of eicosapentaenoic acid in the treatment of atopic dermatitis. A clinical study." *Acta Derm Venereol* (Stockh), 1989;144:139.

195 Berth-Jones, J. & Graham-Brown, R.A.C. "Placebo-controlled trial of essential fatty acid supplementation in atopic dermatitis." *Lancet,* 1993;341:1557–1560.

196 Søyland, E., Funk, J., et al. "Dietary supplementation with very long-chain n-3 fatty acids in patients with atopic dermatitis. A double-blind multicentre study." *Br J Dermatol,* 1994;130:757–764.

197 Poikolainen, K., et al. "Alcohol intake: a risk factor for psoriasis in young and middle aged men?" *BMJ,* 1990;300:780–783.

198 Monk, B.E. & Neill, S.M. "Alcohol consumption and psoriasis." *Dermatologica,* 1986;173:57–60.

199 Douglas, J.M. "Psoriasis and diet." *West J Med,* 1980;133:450.

200 Bittiner, S.B., Tucker, W.F.G., et al. "A double-blind, randomised, placebo-controlled trial of fish oil in psoriasis." *Lancet,* 1988;i:378–380.

201 Kojima, T., Terano, T., et al. "Long-term administration of highly purified eicosapentaenoic acid provides improvement of psoriasis." *Dermatologica,* 1991;182:225–230.

202 Kojima, T, Ternao, T., et al. "Effect of highly purified eicosapentaenoic acid on psoriasis." *J Am Acad Dermatol,* 1989;21:150–151.

203 Dewsbury, E., Graham, P., et al. "Topical eicosapentaenoic acid (EPA) in the treatment of psoriasis." *Br J Dermatol,* 1989;120:581–584.

204 Mayser, P., Mrowietz, U., et al. "W-3 Fatty acid-based lipid infusion in patients with chronic plaque psoriasis: Results of a double-blind, randomized, placebo-controlled, multicenter trial." *J Am Acad Dermatol* 1998;38:539–547.

205 Ashley, J.M., Lowe, N.J., et al. "Fish oil supplementation results in decreased hypertriglyceridemia in patients with psoriasis undergoing etretinate or acitretin therapy." *J Am Acad Dermatol* 1988;19:76–82.

Chapter 8

206 Pizzorno, J., Murray, M., et al. *Clinician's Handbook of Natural Medicine.* London: Churchill Livingstone, 2001: 1519.

207 Kremer, J.M., Jubiz, W., et al. "Fish-oil fatty acid supplementation in active rheumatoid arthritis. A double-blind, controlled, crossover study." *Ann Intern Med,* 1987;106(4):497-503.

208 Cleland, L.G., James, M.J., et al. "Linoleate inhibits EPA incorporation from dietary fish-oil supplements in human subjects." *Am J Clin Nutr,* 1992;55(2):395-399.

209 Geusens, P., Wouters, C., et al. "Long-term effect of omega-3 fatty acid supplementation in active rheumatoid arthritis. A 12-month, double-blind, controlled study." *Arthritis Rheum,* 1994;37(6):824-829.

210 Kremer, J.M., Lawrence, D.A., et al. "Effects of high-dose fish oil on rheumatoid arthritis after stopping nonsteroidal antiinflammatory drugs. Clinical and immune correlates." *Arthritis Rheum,* 1995;38(8):1107-1114.

211 Fortin, P.R., Lew, R.A., et al. "Validation of a meta-analysis: the effects of fish oil in rheumatoid arthritis." *J Clin Epidemiol,* 1995;48(11): 1379-1390.

212 Darlington, L.G. & Stone, T.W. "Antioxidants and fatty acids in the amelioration of rheumatoid arthritis and related disorders." *Br J Nutr,* 2001;85(3):251-269.

213 Kremer, J.M. "N-3 fatty acid supplements in rheumatoid arthritis." *Am J Clin Nutr,* 2000;71(1 Suppl):349S-51S.

214 Shapiro, J.A., et al. "Diet and rheumatoid arthritis in women: a possible protective effect of fish consumption." *Epidemiology,* 1996;7(3):256-263.

215 Kremer, J.M., et al. "Effects of high-dose fish oil on rheumatoid arthritis after stopping nonsteroidal anti-inflammatory drugs. Clinical and immune correlates." *Arthritis and Rheumatism,* 1995;38(8):1107-1114.

216 Lau, C.S., et al. "Effects of fish oil on plasma fibrinolysis in patients with mild rheumatoid arthritis." *Clinical and Experimental Rheumatology,* 1995;13(1):87-90.

Chapter 9

217 Lozano, P., et al. "The economic burden of asthma in US children: estimates from the National Medical Expenditure Survey." *J Allergy Clin Immunol,* 1999;104(5):957-963.

218 Clark, N.M., et al. "Childhood asthma." *Environ Health Perspect,* 1999;107:421-429.

219 Broughton, K.S., et al. "Reduced asthma symptoms with n-3 fatty acid ingestion are related to 5-series leukotriene production." *Am J Clin Nutr,* 1997;65:1011-1017.

220 Hodge, L., et al. "Consumption of oily fish and childhood asthma risk." *MJA,* 1996;164:137-140.

221 Batmanghelidj, F. *ABCs of Asthma, Allergies and Lupus.* Vienna, VA: Global Health Solutions, Inc., 2000.

222 Hodge, L., Salome, C.M., et al. "Consumption of oily fish and childhood asthma risk." *Med J Aust,* 1996;164(3):137-140.

223 Broughton, K.S., Johnson, C.S., et al. "Reduced asthma symptoms with n-3 fatty acid ingestion are related to 5-series leukotriene production." *Am J Clin Nutr,* 1997;65(4):1011-1017.

224 Hashimoto, N., et al. "[Effects of eicosapentaenoic acid in patients with bronchial asthma]." *Nihon Kyobu Shikkan Gakkai Zasshi,* 1997;35(6):634-640.

225 Okamoto, M., et al. "Effects of perilla seed oil supplementation on leukotriene generation by leucocytes in patients with asthma associated with lipometabolism." *International Archives of Allergy and Immunology,* 2000;122(2):137-142.

226 Okamoto, M., et al. "Effects of dietary supplementation with n-3 fatty acids compared with n-6 fatty acids on bronchial asthma." *Intern Med,* 2000;39(2):107-111.

227 Hodge L, Salome CM, Hughes JM, Liu-Brennan D, Rimmer J, Allman M, Pang D, Armour C, Woolcock AJ. Effect of dietary intake of omega-3 and omega-6 fatty acids on severity of asthma in children. *Eur Respir J.* 1998;11(2):361-365.

228 Arm, J.P., Horton, C.E., et al. "The effects of dietary supplementation with fish oil lipids on the airways response to inhaled allergen in bronchial asthma." *Am Rev Respir Dis,* 1989;139(6):1395-1400.

229 Arm JP, Horton CE, et al. "Effect of dietary supplementation with fish oil lipids on mild asthma." *Thorax,* 1988;43(2):84-92.

230 Weiler, J.M. & Ryan, E.J. 3rd. "Asthma in United States olympic athletes who participated in the 1998 olympic winter games." *J Allergy Clin Immunol,* 2000;106(2):267-271.

Chapter 10

231 Seddon, J.M., Rosner, B., et al. "Dietary fat and risk for advanced age-related macular degeneration." *Arch Ophthalmol,* 2001;119(8):1191-1199.

232 Smith, W., Mitchell, P., et al. "Dietary fat and fish intake and age-related maculopathy." *Arch Ophthalmol,* 2000;118(3):401-404.

Chapter 11

233 Mori, T.A., Bao, D.Q., et al. "Dietary fish as a major component of a weight-loss diet: effect on serum lipids, glucose, and insulin metabolism in overweight hypertensive subjects." *Am J Clin Nutr,* 1999;70(5):817-825.

Chapter 12

234 Krajcovicová-Kudláčková, M., et al. "Plasma fatty acid profile and alternative nutrition." *Ann Nutr Metab,* 1997;41(6):365-370.

235 Li, D., et al. "Effect of dietary alpha-linolenic acid on thrombotic risk factors in vegetarian men." *Am J Clin Nutr,* 1999;69(5):872-882.

236 Sanders, T.A., et al. "Essential fatty acid requirements of vegetarians in pregnancy, lactation, and infancy." *Am J Clin Nutr,* 1999;70:555S-559S.

237 Piolot, A., Blache, D., et al. "Effect of fish oil on LDL oxidation and plasma homocysteine concentrations in health." *J Lab Clin Med,* 2003;141(1):41-49.

Appendix C

238 Nutt, D.J., "Discontinuation of Vioxx." *Lancet,* 2005 Jan;365(9453):28.

239 Juni, P., et al. "Risk of cardiovascular events and rofecoxib: Cumulative meta-analysis." *Lancet,* 2004 Dec 4;364(9450):2021-9.

240 Wilde Matthews, A. & Martinez, B. "E-mails suggest Merck knew Vioxx's dangers at early stage." *The Wall Street Journal,* Monday, November 1, 2004:A1.

241 Bjordal, et al. *BMJ,* Nov. 19, 2004 online edition.

242 Bombardier, C., et al. "Comparison of upper gastrointestinal toxicity of rofecoxib and naproxen in patients with rheumatoid arthritis: VIGOR study." *New Engl J Med,* 2000 Nov 3;343(21):1520-8.

243 Richwine, L. "Arthritis drug recall sparks criticism of FDA." Reuters, Monday October 4, 2004.

244 Curtis, C.L., Hughes, C.E., et al. "n-3 fatty acids specifically modulate catabolic factors involved in articular cartilage degradation." *J Biol Chem,* 2000;275(2):721-724.

245 Curtis, C.L., Rees, C.G., et al. "Effects of n-3 fatty acids on cartilate metabolism." *Proc Nutr Soc,* 2002 Aug;61(3):381-9.

246 "Cod liver oil 'slows arthritis.'" BBC News, Thursday, February 4, 2004: http://news.bbc.co.uk/1/hi/health/3480053.stm.

247 Adkisson, H.D., Tranik, T.M., et al. Poster presentation at the Third International Conference on Essential Fatty Acids and Eicosanoids, Adelaide, Australia, 1992 March 1.

248 Curtis, C.L., et al. "Effects of n-3 fatty acids on cartilage metabolism," *Proc Nutr Soc,* 2002 Aug;61(3):381-9.

249 Watkins, B.A., Li, Y., et al. "Minireview: Omega-3 polyunsaturated fatty acids and skeletal health." *Experimental Biology and Medicine,* 2001;226:485-497.

250 James, M.J. & Cleland, L.G. "Dietary n-3 fatty acids and therapy for rheumatoid arthritis." *Semin Arthritis Rheum,* 1997;27:85-97.

251 Adam, O. "Dietary fatty acids and immune reactions in synovial tissue." *Eur J Med Res,* 2003 Aug 20;8(8):381-7.

Appendix D

252 Mann, D. "Natural skin care treatments." Published on WebMD.com; June 5, 2003.

Index

ADHD, *see* Attention Deficit
Disorder/Attention Deficit/Hyperactivity
Disorder
Age-related macular degeneration (AMD),
120-121
ALA, *see* alpha-linolenic acid (ALA)
Albacore, *see* Fish, albacore
Allergies, 25, 31, 34, 84, 103, 106,
108, 116, 164
to food—72, 108
in relation to ADHD, 80
Alpha-linolenic acid (ALA), 13, 49-50, 81,
97-98, 113, 127, 136, 152, 159-160
AMD, *see* Age-related macular
degeneration (AMD)
Angina, 40, 46
Antidepressants, *see* Medications
Antioxidants, 33, 59, 69-70, 112,
120, 134-136
synthetic—21
Arthritis, 15, 17, 20, 26, 28-29, 84, 108-113,
125, 146-155, 164, 146-155, 164
see also Osteoarthritis,
Rheumatoid arthritis
Asthma, 80-81, 119, 139
Attention Deficit Disorder/Attention
Deficit/Hyperactivity Disorder, 16, 71-86,
91, 109, 151

Baby formulas, 16, 73, 91
Barlean's Fishery, 145
Beef, 58, 82, 97, 131
see also Meats

Behavioral disorders, 32, 34, 62, 64, 67, 68,
71-72, 75-76, 78, 81-83, 86, 101
see also Attention Deficit
Disorder/Attention Deficit/Hyperactivity
Disorder
Bipolar disorders, 68-69, 75
Blood clots, 6, 14, 45, 126, 162
Brain development, 5-6, 13, 16, 20, 32,
45, 62, 64, 66, 73-75, 78-79, 81, 83, 87,
89-93
Breast milk, 16, 18, 72-73, 87-93
Butter, 22, 27, 110, 118

Cancer
breast—20, 22, 49-57, 103
colon—15, 50-51, 55-56
colorectal—54, 55
lung—52-53, 58
pancreatic—58, 60
prostate—20, 52-53, 56
rectal—32, 51, 55-56
Carbohydrates, 17, 25, 66, 72, 80,
85, 94-95, 99, 122, 135
Carrots, *see* vegetables
Cells
membranes of—82-84, 90, 96, 101,
105, 109
red blood—14, 41, 61-62, 65-66,
92-93, 126
structure of—17, 64, 82
white blood—110, 115-117
Cholesterol, 6, 14, 17-18, 20, 41-42, 44, 45,
63-64, 82, 90, 95-99, 117, 121, 123,
136, 140, 151-152, 154-155
HDL—1, 123, 154
LDL—45, 98, 117, 136, 154

Cod liver oil, 45, 66, 136, 142-143, 152-153
Coenzyme Q_{10} (CoQ_{10}), 44
Cooking methods
  baking—2
  boiling—58
  frying—20, 30, 58, 86, 97
CoQ_{10}, see Coenzyme$_{10}$ (CoQ_{10})
COX-2 inhibitors, 146-155
Custom canned albacore, see Fish, albacore

Depression, 7, 16, 62-66, 75, 78, 83, 88,
  103, 125, 164
  postpartum—88, 91
DHA (docosahexanaic acid), 6, 11-14, 16,
  19, 27, 32, 37, 40-41, 44, 46, 49-52, 58,
  63-67, 69, 72-73, 81-84, 86-93, 98, 104,
  109-110, 112-113, 117-118, 126, 135,
  136, 145, 152, 154, 159-160
Diabetes, 15, 17, 20, 22-23, 26, 29,
  45, 94-100, 124, 136, 139, 151, 159,
  162, 164
Docosahexanaic acid, see DHA
  (docosahexanaic acid)
Dysmenorrhea, 104

Eczema, 80, 103-106, 125,
  156-157, 160, 164
EFAs, see Essential fatty acids (EFAs)
Eicosapentaenoic acid, see EPA
  (eicosapentaenoic acid)
EPA (eicosapentaenoic acid), 6, 11, 12, 13,
  19, 40, 41, 44, 46, 49-69, 81, 84, 88,
  90, 98-99, 102-110, 115-121, 135-136,
  152-154, 159-160
Essential fatty acids (EFAs), 19-21, 27, 80,
  81, 105, 153
Exercise, 42-43, 46, 56, 95, 99, 119,
  122-123, 133
Eyes, 5-6, 65, 73, 81, 85, 120-121
  see also Age-related macular degeneration
  (AMD)
Fish
  albacore—11, 130-132
  farm-raised—27, 37, 128
  salmon—11-12, 21, 24, 37, 70, 100,
  115-116, 124, 132, 145
  tuna—11-13, 16, 20-21, 23-24, 27, 30,
  32, 47, 53, 70, 72, 79, 82, 85, 91, 96-98,
  100, 118, 124, 130-132

Fish oils, 6, 11, 14-16, 23-24, 28, 38-41,
  44,46, 50-51, 58, 66, 85, 92, 97-98,
  109-110, 112, 128-129, 136, 142-155,
  160, 163
  in supplement form—13, 15, 25, 33, 37,
  39, 45-47, 60, 66, 67, 69, 81, 85, 90
  pharmaceutical quality of—13, 129, 136,
  142-143
  purity of—131, 135, 143
Flaxseed, 12-13, 17, 19, 21, 23, 26, 33,
  57-58, 66, 82, 86-87, 99, 113, 122,
  124-128, 135, 145, 156, 160, 162

Gamma-linolenic acid, 102-105
Grains, 22, 26, 30, 99, 125, 135, 156

Hair health, 103, 105, 125, 156, 158,
  163-164
HDL, see High density lipoproteins (HDL)
Heart disease, 6, 14, 20-23, 26, 28-30,
  37-38, 40, 43, 45, 47, 63, 122, 126,
  138-140, 154-155, 158-162, 164
High blood pressure, 14, 17, 41-43, 92, 94,
  97-99, 123
High density lipoproteins (HDL), 6, 14,
  41, 154
Hydrogenated oils, 22-23, 25-27, 33,
  104, 118
Hyperactivity, see ADHD
Hypertension, 22, 41-44, 123, see also High
  blood pressure

Iceland
  health conditions in—5-7
Iceland Health, Inc., 142-143
Icelandic Longevity Institute, 6
Infants, 5, 7, 16, 31, 65, 72, 83, 87, 89-93,
  114, 126
Inflammatory diseases, 6, 20, 28-29, 65, 84,
  105, 109, 112, 113-114, 147-155, 157,
  159, 160-162, 164
Insulin, 94-99, 122-123, 135, 162

Joints
  effects of omega-3 on—6, 11, 13, 15,
  111, 149, 153-155
  effects of poor diet on—125
  inflammation—20, 23, 108
  see also Arthritis

Kidneys, 15, 20, 32, 41, 94, 96, 102, 149

LDL, *see* Low density lipoproteins (LDL)
Liver, 15, 89
Low density lipoproteins (LDL), 6, 14, 45,
    97-99, 117, 123, 136, 154
Lupus, 20, 28

Margarine, 21-23, 110, 118
Meats, 7, 19, 20, 30, 54, 56, 59, 109, 112,
    124-125, 130-131, 140, 159
    chicken—27, 30, 123, 131
    free-range livestock—12, 131
    grain-fed—59, 109, 113
Medications
    Adderall—74, 76, 78
    anti-inflammatory—6, 15, 26, 52, 108,
    111-112
    Celebrex—147-148, 150
    Lexapro—74
    nitroglycerin—46
    Ritalin—24, 71-72, 74-78, 81, 85
    Vioxx—147-151
    Zoloft—75
Menopause, 103
Menstruation, 102, 104
Mental Health, 62-63, 65-67

NSAIDs (Non-steroidal anti-inflammatory
    drugs), *see* Medications,
    anti-inflammatory

Obesity, 14, 22, 29, 94-96, 99, 122-123,
    134, 139

Olde World Icelandic Cod Liver Oil™, 51, 143
Omega-3 fatty acids, 44-86, 90, 92, 98-99,
    102-105, 109-113, 115-129, 132-133,
    135, 138-141, 146-164
Omega-6 fatty acids, 7, 12 19-22, 24-34,
    38-52, 56, 59, 63, 65, 67, 69, 73, 82-83,
    90-91, 97-98, 101, 105, 109-110,
    112-115, 120-121, 125-127, 134-135,
    146-147, 149, 153-155
Organic foods, 22, 56, 134
    beef—130
    flax seed—127-128
    milk and yogurt—99
    vegetables—134-135
Osteoarthritis, 108, 112, 146-147, 149-152
Osteoporosis, 102, 124

PMS, *see* Postmenstrual Syndrome
Postmenstrual Syndrome (PMS), 101, 103
Pregnancy, 13-14, 17-18, 41, 47, 65-66,
    87-89, 91-93, 101, 116
Prostaglandins, 6, 18, 20, 25, 48, 52, 65,
    80-81, 101, 104-105, 108-109, 112, 113,
    149-150, 154, 156
Psoriasis, 103-107, 125, 157

Rheumatoid arthritis, 15, 17, 28, 108,
    110-113, 149-152, 154-155

Salmon, *see* Fish, salmon
Seafood, 13-14, 23, 33, 37, 47, 66, 68,
    87, 132
    see also Fish
Serotonin, 16, 63, 83, 91, 151
Skin health, 6, 11, 12, 16, 69, 80, 104-106,
    125, 130, 157-164
Stroke, 5, 14, 20, 23, 26, 29, 37, 45, 94,
    122, 125, 126, 147-150, 152, 159, 161
Sun
    protection from with omega-3s—162
Syndrome X, 95-99

Triglycerides, 6, 14-15, 45, 94, 99, 107, 117,
    123, 155

Vegetable Oils, 12, 19, 23, 26-31, 33, 49, 97,
    106, 109-110, 118, 127, 130, 135, 159
    canola—19
    corn—20, 26, 28, 82, 111, 117-118
    olive—18, 22, 33, 51, 58-59, 68, 110,
    118, 122
Vegetable Shortening, 23, 27
Vegetables, 12, 19, 22, 26, 42, 44, 53, 63,
    95, 99, 134, 135
    carrots—53, 135
Vitamins, 25, 66-68, 86, 103, 134-136,
    142-143, 155, 159, 161-162
    A—136, 143
    B$_{12}$—116, 136
    C—44, 95, 112, 135
    D—102, 143
    E—39, 46, 60-61, 69, 85, 112, 135, 136

Weight loss, 42-43, 60, 64, 74, 95, 122-123

About the Authors

Garry Gordon, M.D., D.O., M.D.(H.), received his Doctor of Osteopathy in 1958 from the Chicago College of Osteopathy in Illinois. He received his honorary M.D. degree from the University of California, Irvine in 1962 and completed his Radiology Residency from Mt. Zion in San Francisco, California in 1964. For many years, he was the Medical Director of Mineral Lab in Hayward, California, a leading laboratory for trace mineral analysis worldwide.

Dr. Gordon is on the Board of Homeopathic Medical Examiners for Arizona and is cofounder of the American College for Advancement in Medicine (ACAM). He is founder/president of the International College of Advanced Longevity (ICALM) and board member of International Oxidative Medicine Association (IOMA).

With Morton Walker, D.P.M., Dr. Gordon co-authored *The Chelation Answer.* He is advisor to the American Board of Chelation Therapy and past instructor and examiner for all chelation physicians. He is responsible for Peer Review for Chelation Therapy in the State of Arizona.

Currently, Dr. Gordon is a full-time consultant for Longevity Plus, a nutritional supplement company located in Payson, Arizona. He is responsible for the design of the majority of their supplements, which are widely used by alternative health practitioners around the world. Dr. Gordon can be reached by calling (928) 472-4263 or through his website *www.gordonresearch.com.*

Herb Joiner-Bey, N.D., is an experienced primary-care natural health practitioner, specializing in classical homeopathy, therapeutic nutrition, Western botanical medicine, and the conventional treatment of sexually transmitted diseases. He places strong focus on emotional, social, and spiritual aspects of healing. He is also a dynamic professional educator and seminar leader who has trained thousands of health care professionals in the philosophy and clinical application of modern, scientifically verified natural medicine. Dr. Bey is the author of several books, a CD-ROM, and numerous articles in this field. In addition, he serves as medical/scientific editor for several journals and magazines focused on integrative medicine. He is an adjunct professor of classical homeopathy and advanced therapeutics at Bastyr University, Kenmore, Washington, and a consultant to several manufacturers of the highest-quality products in the nutriceutical/health food industry. He also serves as guest speaker on natural medicine for radio talk shows across the nation. Dr. Bey holds a B.A. degree in physics from Johns Hopkins University, Baltimore, Maryland, and an N.D. (Doctor of Naturopathic Medicine) degree from Bastyr University.